LIFE IS HOW YOU TELL YOUR STORY

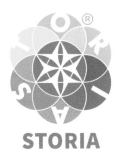

STORIA

LIFE IS HOW YOU TELL YOUR STORY

A MOTHER'S QUEST TO HEAL HER SON

Written by Yamina Salomon
Edited by Audrey Serper

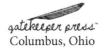

gatekeeper press™
Columbus, Ohio

Life Is How You Tell Your Story: A Mother's Quest to Heal Her Son

Published by Gatekeeper Press
2167 Stringtown Rd, Suite 109
Columbus, OH 43123-2989
www.GatekeeperPress.com

Library of Congress Control Number: 2021944342
ISBN (paperback): 9781662909351
eISBN: 9781662909368

Book Front Cover: Arieldavid's portrait of his future self at age twenty-one, painted when he was eleven by Massimo Pedrazzi in 2017.

Photograph Credits: Yamina Salomon and by Karina Glikin Yarri

Disclaimer:

Although the information contained in this book is based on true events, it should not be taken as a recommendation for treatment. For any medical condition, always consult with a qualified physician.

The author of this book does not determine, guarantee, or qualify the competence of any person listed in this book. The use of this book to locate and engage with persons listed in the book is at the reader's own risk.

The information and other content provided in this book, or in any linked materials, is for informational purposes only and is not intended as medical advice. Readers are encouraged to consult directly with their medical providers on their specific needs.

Contact Info:

To get in touch with the author of this book, feel free to contact Yamina at her website, STORIAMAP.COM, or via her email yamina@storiamap.com.

This Book Is Dedicated...

To my mother, Atalia Salomon, who never gave up on me, even when she was facing challenges after my father was killed in the Yom Kippur War, and to her life partner, Jeff Belman. Thank you both for being there for me and Arieldavid, no matter what.

To the memory of my grandparents, Ada and Shimon Nachmani, for loving me unconditionally and teaching me how to imagine solutions to any challenge. You all are my role models for what motherhood is all about.

To the memory of Adam Fish, to Moshe Fibich, and to Rachel Ben Ari. Thank you for your bravery in standing up for what is just. Thank you for the six-year-long, pro-bono, court battle you won so that Arieldavid could live at home like any other child. I will remember and be thankful to you, always.

To all mothers, wherever and whoever you are—know that I truly believe in the power of motherhood, a power you hold within yourself. It is the power of cocreation! I know from my own experience as a mother: if you believe and do your part, the impossible becomes possible!

Contents

Special Thanks

Gratitude goes to a long list of people that assisted me with the creation of this book. But there are four people to whom I am especially grateful for being in my life, and without them, this book would never have reached your hands.

The first one is Audrey, who has been a true friend for more than twelve years and was a witness to my life's challenges and the actions I took in order to create the life I dreamed of for my son and me. Audrey believed in me and in the contribution to other mothers this story would bring. She encouraged me to write this book and to share the things I've learned. Audrey shaped the words of this book with much attention and dedication, and even in the busiest time of her own life, she still continued to do this with the same intent in heart: to do her best to make this book clear and helpful to the reader. Thank you with all my heart, Audrey, for your help and for being a true friend every step of the way.

The second person is my mom, Atalia Salomon, who, thanks to her ongoing support, enabled me to make this journey in the first place. You supported me in all the years of hardship. You taught me not to give up and to continue looking for solutions. And with your beautiful laughter at the end of an encouraging conversation, you would remind me that life is too short to be wasted on negativity and should rather be enjoyed. You are a role model for what motherhood is truly all about: believing in your child and supporting him, no matter what. I love you, Mom.

The third person is my guru, Dr. Jayant Kumar Bhadury, my *Bhrigu* yoga teacher since 2012, who teaches me how to live a balanced life. Thank you for your dedication, patience, and care. You are a role model in understanding how the body and mind can be used to create purity and balance in life. Thank you for being my teacher, guide, and a good example to follow.

And last but not least, thank you to my beloved son, Arieldavid. Without you, this journey would not have taken place to begin with. You are my biggest teacher, and it is thanks to you that I have entered into the yoga, Ayurveda, and yoga therapy worlds to awaken to my own internal powers, born out of my unconditional love for you. I believe in you, kid! Thank you for choosing me to be your mom.

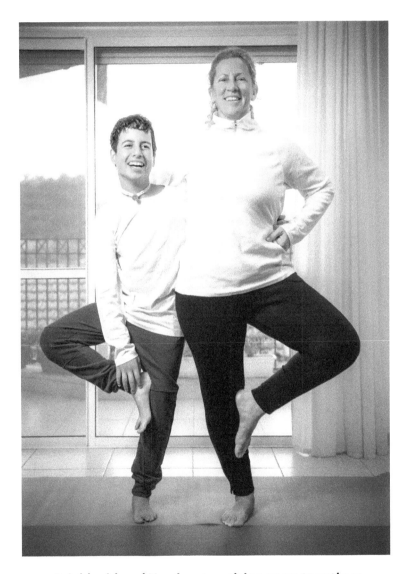

Arieldavid and Yamina practicing yoga together:
Tree Pose/Vriksasana, 2020

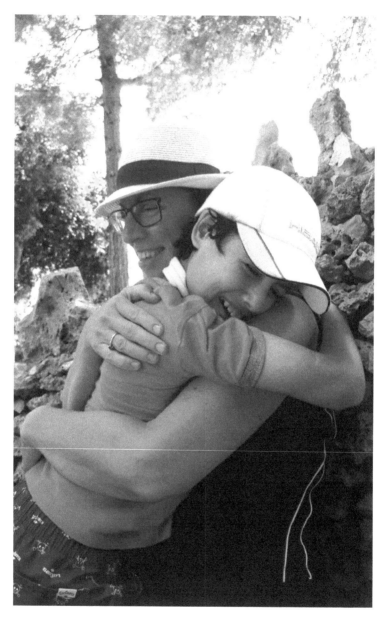

Arieldavid and Yamina, 2018

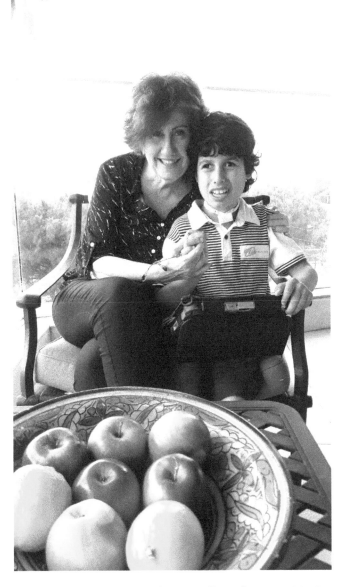

Arieldavid and Grandma Atalia Salomon, 2018

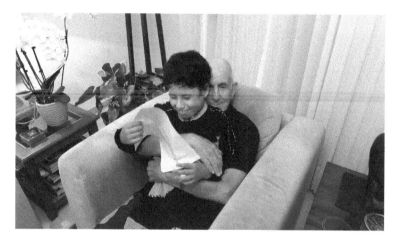

Arieldavid and Grandpa Jeff Belman, 2018

Introduction

The rain is pouring hard outside my window as I am writing these words. This is a significant moment for me. I have been waiting for so long to begin writing this book, for more than ten years. It is symbolic for me to write the beginning of my story while it is raining. The rain is a symbol of my wish, the wish that this book will wash and purify our negative emotions, limiting belief systems, and thought patterns, and will ultimately lead to the necessary changes in our behavior that will allow us to have a healthy, happy, and balanced life. The rain is a natural *Shodhana* (purification) process as it purifies the air we breathe. Normally, most of us, myself included, do not really think about these things in our daily lives as we rush to take our kids to school in the morning or rush to work while trying our best to avoid the traffic. We do not normally think: "Ah! It is raining. Rain purifies. We are now breathing clean air." We just take it for granted, just as we take for granted every breath we take—it's automatic, so we do not really think about it.

But this book is not about rushing, nor is it about taking things for granted. On the contrary, this book is about stopping our automatic behavior and starting to think about things that do matter to us, such as what makes us feel joy, love and happiness. It is about contemplating why we do what we do through *Svadhyaya* (self-study). It is where we develop a sense of curiosity about ourselves, our thought patterns, beliefs, behaviors, emotions, and overall interaction with others, the environment, and life itself. This book is also about making choices that are born out of a deeper calling, from the intention to sanctify life and live in *Santosha* (contentment).

I wrote this book out of my personal experience as a mother to a beautiful young man called Arieldavid. Arieldavid was born with a rare, life-threatening disease called Haddad syndrome. Today, against all odds, my son is fifteen years old and enjoys a full and beautiful life. He goes horseback riding once a week, bicycles with me or his dad once or twice a week, and walks in nature almost every day. Arieldavid goes to school regularly and is a loved student by his classmates and teachers. At home he loves to help in the kitchen and makes healthy chocolate balls from dates and hazelnuts. He also waters the plants in the garden every morning after he feeds the neighborhood cats. Every morning, we practice yoga, which we have done since he was five years old.

I am sharing this with you not to brag but to say that the impossible is possible. If you saw him today, you would not think that what we went through happened, but it did.

As I observed my son develop and grow out of the traumatic events connected with the chronic condition he was born with, I felt inspired to share the knowledge I intuitively gained and later on expanded with professional studies of the body, mind, and emotions. This includes studying *Ayurveda* for three years on Broshim Campus, becoming a registered integrated yoga teacher in 2011, and a journey practitioner certified by Brandon Bays in 2020. I have studied *Bhrigu* yoga for over nine years with Dr. Bhadury and still continue to study under his guidance. Most recently, I have been studying yoga therapy with Mrs. Zipi Negev, which I will be completing in 2021.

This book tells my personal story, but it may also be used as a self-help guidebook as I provide various examples, exercises, and teachings from yoga philosophy, *Ayurveda*, and the Storia Method that I developed. The examples and knowledge stem from my personal practice with my son as well as from my experience as a yoga teacher and a Storia meditation and visualization instructor.

This book is a testimony to the power of belief, imagination, and love. It is a testimony to how children can do the impossible if only you believe in them. When you believe in your children and support them throughout their journey, you give them a real chance to grow and realize themselves. This book will show you how you can transform unthinkable pain into an opportunity to see the beauty in life in all its glory. How you can connect to your inner light, tapping into the God spark within you, and learn to navigate yourself effectively to a place of curiosity, joy, and fulfillment.

This book may motivate you to help yourself and your children to live from a place of love and dedication; to let go of the pain and the harmful habits while embracing happiness and well-being in your life, while helping others to embrace it as well.

I hope that by reading this book you will see that children born with chronic health conditions are our saviors, our wake-up call as they challenge us to become better people. They challenge us to be more responsible in our relationships with ourselves, our families, our communities, and the world around us. They improve us because their pain propels us to become better, and their healing helps to heal our hearts, making the world we live in a little bit better.

I wrote this book for parents, caregivers, teachers, social workers, nurses, doctors, and therapists with the intention of bringing peace and hope and inspiring you to believe in yourself and give you the tools to reach your dreams and help others as well.

"Lady," said the Emperor, when Fatima was brought before him, "Can you make a tent?" "I think so," said Fatima. She asked for rope, but there was none

to be had. So, remembering her time as a spinner, she collected flax and made ropes. Then she asked for stout cloth, but the Chinese had none of the kind she needed. So, drawing on her experience with the weavers of Alexandria, she made some stout tent cloth. Then she found that she needed tent-poles, but there were none in China. So Fatima, remembering how she had been trained by the wood fashioner of Istanbul, made stout tent-poles. When these were ready, she racked her brains for the memory of all the tents she had seen in her travels: and a tent was made. When this wonder was revealed to the Emperor of China, he offered Fatima the fulfilment of any wish she cared to name. She chose to settle in China, where she married a handsome prince and remained in happiness, surrounded by her children, until the end of her days.

–Fatima the Spinner and the Tent,
Tales of the Dervishes, *by Idries Shah*

CHAPTER 1
"Sanctify Life!"

If one advances confidently in the direction of his dreams, and endeavors to live the life which he has imagined, he will meet with a success unexpected in common hours.

–Walden *by Henry David Thoreau*

"Sanctify life!"

"Sanctify life!"

"Sanctify life!"

These were the words that echoed in my mind as I was meditating, gazing at a beautiful oak tree a few meters from my house. I had never meditated before this moment. "Sanctify life!" The words kept echoing inside me. I was gazing at the tree with such focus and intensity that I lost any notion of time and space, and for a few long minutes, I was completely one with that old, big, and beautiful oak tree that was in front of my house outside of my garden.

I hadn't noticed that tree till that very day, when I returned from the hospital and sat down, overwhelmed by the news the doctor had given me. Just a few hours earlier, I was sitting in front of the doctor for a check-up two weeks before my son was born.

"Something is wrong with the baby," the doctor blurted out without any warning. "I recommend you have an abortion."

Shocked by this sudden turn of events, I could not fully comprehend what she was saying. *Everything was going so well. How did this happen?* I thought. *And how could she suggest I have an abortion?!* I was shocked as, for me, this soon-to-be-born baby was a gift from God, which I had no intention of turning down. At that point in time, it was not even clear exactly what the problem was.

"What are you talking about?!" I replied. "Abortion? No way! I love my son, and I want him to live! And if he is sick, which you don't even know for certain, you don't even know what the sickness is. But should this be the case, what I want from you as a doctor is to help him live and to guide me in how to help him heal!"

Now, it was the doctor who looked surprised. But seeing that my mind and heart were aligned in a firm answer, all she could do was nod. "I will arrange a meeting with the relevant doctors," she said, "so that your son will receive the necessary life support on the day of his birth."

I returned home, feeling overwhelmed but knowing I had done the right thing. I felt a big storm was coming my way, and I was not sure how to approach it. *What is our life going to be like?* I asked myself as I sat down in my living room, overlooking the garden.

My gaze fell naturally to an old oak tree, and as if nothing else existed, I was drawn to observe it. I saw the strong and stable tree trunk. It seemed like nothing could ever move it. I wanted to be as strong as that trunk, regardless of what the doctor had said. I wanted to follow my own heart. I knew intuitively that my son would be healed. There was no explanation for that internal "knowing," but I felt, with all my heart, that this baby would grow to be as strong and beautiful as this oak tree.

"God will prevail, and he will help us in our journey," I said to myself.

I looked up at the tree's leaves. The wind was moving them in all directions. These leaves were swirling and crackling just like my thoughts, making me restless. I shifted my gaze back to the tree trunk and again regained calmness and balance as the sturdiness I was witnessing was reflected back into my own soul. My gaze became stronger, and I felt closer to the tree, as if I were just a few meters away from it. I began breathing with the tree, inhaling cold air and exhaling warm air from my body. Slowly I felt my breath becoming deeper and steadier.

This tree has seen extreme weather, storms and even wars, I thought to myself. *And yet it is still standing strong and beautiful, looking so majestic and wise.* I felt as if I was standing right beside it. I imagined myself leaning on it, putting my arms around it, and letting go. Feeling all the burdens leaving me, feeling grounded, feeling at peace.

I turned to the tree and asked it, "Tell me what path I should take." I was talking to the tree without any expectations of receiving an answer. But the answer did come. I could hear the words in my mind, as clear as day:

"Sanctify life!"

"Sanctify life!"

The words were still echoing in my head. I wanted to help my son live the best life he could. I didn't exactly know how I would do this, but now I had a path: "sanctify life."

Note*: Thirteen years later I call this meditation "Storia's tree meditation" and use it in my Storia Map workshops. You will find the script for Storia's tree meditation in the upcoming pages, so you may practice it too. The main benefit you may attain, as I have, is to find the core value of your life, your own personal mantra.*

The Dream and the Promise to My Son

Two weeks later I had a dream.

In the dream, I heard a noise in the hallway of my home, so I walked to the entrance door. The door opened, and a stranger walked in. He stopped and stood in front of me. To my surprise, I was not scared. The man's face was incredibly peaceful. I knew he had not come to harm me.

"Are you lost? Do you need something? A glass of water?" I asked the man in the dream. He was taller than me, but not by much, and he had short silver hair. His body was slim yet strong. I felt very calm.

He shook his head as if to say, "No, I am not lost. I have come to the right place." He lifted his right hand and rested it ever so softly on his chest. He bowed his head slightly as if to say, "I apologize if I startled you and came uninvited."

"I am not startled," I answered, "but if you are not lost, why did you come?"

My mind was racing with questions, but strangely, my body was completely relaxed. We were only one meter away from each other. The man was now facing forward, looking straight into my eyes. His eyes were light blue. *Such beautiful eyes,* I thought to myself. *There is so much PEACE in them.* Peace I had not seen before in anyone's eyes. This peace was so vivid and distinct in contrast to the turbulence I was experiencing in my life. In contrast to the stress, the running around and worrying, these eyes were like a safe harbor on a stormy night. It was as if his eyes were calling out like a lighthouse sending a beacon to the ships at sea, showing them the way back home.

I stood there with my feet firmly on the ground and looked straight ahead into the man's eyes, waiting for his answer.

"Everything will be all right." His words were very clear and sharp, cutting all illusions of uncertainty. I understood. He had come to give me an encouraging message. To give me the strength I needed to help my son live.

"Yes, I know," I said. "But how can I help him?"

At that very moment, I woke up. It was around five in the morning. My water broke, and I rushed to the hospital to give birth to my son. He was a beautiful baby, and when I looked at him, I only saw beautiful, emanating light.

The day Arieldavid was born, I held his tiny hand in mine. I leaned close to his beautiful face and whispered to him softly, with confidence, "I promise you, you will have an amazing life, no matter what. I will do everything in my power to help you heal and have a happy, full life! Don't worry. Mom is always with you!"

To this very day, I lovingly fulfill the promise I made to my son fifteen years ago at the hospital on the day he was born. I do this with *Mudita*, which in Sanskrit means "The joy that comes out of being happy in another person's happiness." Thus, it makes me happy to see my son happy.

Note: *A few years later, I was attending a retreat for the Sacred Movement in Nocera Umbra, Italy. And as I entered the Monastery San Biagio, where the retreat was being held, there he was, the man from my dream. "Is this possible?" I thought to myself. "Could this really be the same man? Did he extend his consciousness and communicate with me through my dream? If this is possible, there would be so many advantages to having this ability, so many new possibilities to help others."*

He greeted me with "Benvenuti," meaning "Welcome" in Italian. If it was really him, I never got a chance to thank him personally for the gift he gave me that night, the strength, and affirmation through a simple message: "Everything will be okay."

I continued to ponder as I walked in and internally said to him, "I thank you, Signor G."

The First Months of My Son's Life

In the last decade, epigenetic research has
established that DNA blueprints passed down
through genes are not set in concrete at birth.
Genes are not destiny! Environmental influences,
including nutrition, stress, and emotions,
can modify those genes...
—The Biology of Belief *by Bruce H. Lipton*

In 2005, Arieldavid was born and was immediately connected to a ventilation machine that kept him alive. Within days of his delivery, it was already apparent that we were not going home any time soon. In the beginning the doctors still were not exactly sure what the problem was. This gave us an advantage, since the doctors were always around, constantly on alert, ready to treat Arieldavid with the best of care. Within a couple of days, after various tests, they were able to give a diagnosis. My son was diagnosed with Haddad syndrome, which was a surprise to the doctors, who had expected something completely different.

The doctors informed me that Haddad syndrome is a very rare disease, with only a few documented cases. At the time of Arieldavid's birth, only around thirty-two case studies from around the world had been documented, providing very little information, as the case studies were scarce and seemed to be diverse and inconsistent. However, what was known was that Haddad syndrome was characterized by a combination of two major syndromes—CCHS (Congenital Central Hypoventilation Syndrome) and HD (Hirschsprung Disease). CCHS is a rare genetic neurological disorder that affects the nerves that control involuntary body functions. As a result, babies born with CCHS usually don't have the capacity to breathe on their own and have to be ventilated from birth during the night hours and, in more severe cases, throughout the day as well.

HD is a genetic disorder characterized by the absence of particular nerve cells (ganglions) in the bowel, which damages the ability to move stool through the intestines, leading to partial or total constipation. I was told that this might lead to discomfort and even pain. Little did I know the extent of the pain and suffering I would witness my son go through in the first few years of his life because of this disorder.

The doctors explained that if this disorder was not treated in time, a serious bacterial infection might develop. The specific symptoms can vary from one person to another. In order to enable proper digestion, surgery is needed, in which the part of the intestine that has no ganglions is removed. This operation is called Soave and is considered to be complicated.

Once the diagnosis was given, within a month of Arieldavid's birth, he was scheduled for two major operations. The first was the Soave operation as described above, and the second was called a tracheostomy operation, related to the CCHS, which would allow my son to be connected to a ventilation machine through the trachea—the air canal. Tracheostomy is considered to be an invasive form of ventilation.

Basically, there are two forms of home ventilation; one is invasive—with a tube through an incision in the throat— and the other is noninvasive, with a mask over the mouth and nose. There are different reasons and advantages for both forms of ventilations. Choosing either one is not an easy decision to make.

In AD's case, I wanted very much to choose a noninvasive form of ventilation for him; this meant a face mask or a nose and mouth mask that would be connected to the ventilation machine. This type of ventilation is typically chosen for individuals that need the ventilation machine only at night. But since AD needed to be ventilated during all the hours of the day as well, we were advised to go with the invasive form of ventilation, because it is connected directly to the windpipe through a small hole in the throat, freeing up the face, allowing my son to eat freely and be engaged with people around him and enjoy the environment without a mask barrier.

However, there are two major disadvantages to using the tracheostomy tube. The first is that it puts the individual at constant threat of suffocation that may lead to death if the tube is blocked or removed without an alternative way to ventilate. The second disadvantage is that the tracheostomy tube is situated under the vocal cords. This means that the air needed to produce sound diverts, and instead of moving up through the vocal cords, it moves out through the tracheostomy tube, making it very difficult to create coherent sounds, inhibiting a person's ability to speak.

During the first month of his life, AD suffered much pain waiting for these operations. Unfortunately, he suffered much pain after the operations as well, because the Soave surgery proved to be only partially successful, resulting in many incidents and hospitalizations in the future.

As the days went by in the hospital, I encouraged my son not to give up and told him that things would improve. I would hold him close to my chest and whisper loving words softly in his ear. I would tell him how much I loved him and that I would always be by his side, forever.

I would tell him how wonderful he was, how brave, and how proud I was to be his mother. I described to him the beautiful world that was waiting for him to explore and be a part of. I quickly became very involved with his hospitalization and began to do whatever I could and was allowed to do to help take care of him.

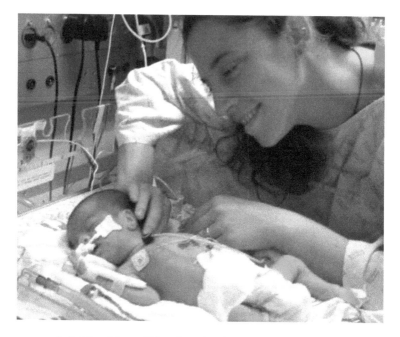

Arieldavid and Yamina in the ICU, shortly after
Arieldavid's birth, 2005

I did not leave my son's bedside. When it came to treatments, I regularly pleaded with the doctors to check Arieldavid's abilities before deciding on his fate based on the few examples described in the textbooks. Some doctors were rigid and unwilling to change, but others were more open and flexible, and thanks to their kind heart and patience, we were even able to avoid unnecessary surgery. Apparently, in medical books dating from the early eighties, it was reported that individuals with Haddad syndrome sometimes have an additional problem with swallowing food. For this reason, it was documented in the medical books that swallowing food was not possible for these individuals and surgery was needed to make a hole in the stomach to feed them directly via an external tube.

But I knew that my son was able to swallow. I could see that there was no saliva coming out of his mouth while he was sucking on the ventilation tube connected to his mouth. I shared my observations with the doctors, but that was not enough evidence for them to be convinced that the cases in the textbook were unrelated to my son's case.

So, for the next few days, I pleaded with the doctors to conduct an experiment to verify once and for all if Arieldavid could swallow or not. They were reluctant to do it because there was a risk of food entering the air canal. I argued that if we did it with only a minute portion of food, it would not harm my son and would be worth the risk because it would eliminate not only an additional surgery but also a lifelong battle to live with a feeding tube that would be hard to manage along with being ventilated.

"He will pass the test!" I said to the doctors. "Just give him a chance."

One night, when it was peaceful and quiet in the ICU, one doctor agreed to help me. She was a kind and gentle doctor, who talked softly to Arieldavid, and he responded to her gentleness and cooperated fully. He passed the test with flying colors, and it was clear to all that he could swallow as he drank from the bottle of my own milk that I was keeping for him in the refrigerator.

Witnessing the agonizing pain my son went through during his first four months of life as he struggled to live, I felt a deep need to get him out of the hospital as fast as I could and continue to help him from home. However, for a ventilated baby with a serious problem in the colon, treatment from home was a significant, life-changing decision strongly advised against by the doctors. The doctors told me I didn't have to do this, that there were places Arieldavid could be put in. But I knew in my heart that those places were not suitable for us. I wanted my son to be with me at home and to raise him like a normal child.

Once the doctors saw I was determined to take Arieldavid home, they began to prepare me for the medical implications of this big step and taught me the medical aspects I would need to know in order to manage his health in the best way.

Over the following several days, the chief nurse taught me all the necessary procedures, including how to operate and maintain all of Arieldavid's manual and electric medical equipment, how to monitor his vital signs and other important physiological parameters, how and when to change the tracheostomy tube and the tracheostomy belt, how to perform tracheostomy suctioning to remove clogged-up mucus, and how to perform resuscitation in case of suffocation or breath-holding spells, as well as what to do in case of other emergencies.

After four months in the neonatal ICU, Arieldavid was discharged from the hospital. I was so relieved to finally leave the hospital and so happy to go home with my son.

My Sadhana as a Young Mother

Practice is the continuous struggle to become firmly established in the stable state of the True Self.

–Yoga Sutras of Patanjali, I, 13

Sadhana is a Sanskrit word that means daily spiritual practice, but it is much more than just a daily routine. Sadhana is a platform with which you help yourself to take charge of your life. It is in the Sadhana *where you become a navigator to your own happiness, longevity, and the cocreator to the story you want to live.*

In her book The Path of Practice, a Woman's Book of Ayurvedic Healing, *Bri. Maya Tiwari describes* Sadhana *as "practices encompass all our daily activities from the simple to the sublime—from cooking a meal to exploring your inner self through meditation."*

Tiwari explains that the word Sadhana derives from the root: "Sadh, which means to reclaim that which is divine in us, our power to heal, serve, rejoice, and uplift the spirit." She writes that the goal of Sadhana is: "To enable you to recover your natural rhythms and realign your inner life and daily habits with the cycles of the universe. When you begin to live and move with the rhythms of nature, your mind becomes more lucid and more peaceful, and your health improves. Your entire life becomes easier."

From my own perspective, when you take on your Sadhana, you are basically saying: "I am willing and worthy of having a healthy body and mind," or "I love myself in a healthy way." The Sadhana is a relationship with your higher self and with God. The Sadhana is the place where one heals, purifies, improves, strengthens, and energize one's body, mind, and spirit.

My own Sadhana continuously develops to this day, and it touches on all aspects of my life, my daily routine, cooking, my profession, my hobbies, my values, and more.

When my son was born, I wasn't yet familiar with the term Sadhana. However, I had my personal mantra, "cherish life," and at that point in time, it meant keeping my son alive and helping him grow. That was my Sadhana, my daily spiritual practice.

Once we went home from the hospital, my daily routine for almost eight years consisted of twenty-four to thirty-six waking hour cycles every forty-eight hours. During the day, I made sure Arieldavid was properly ventilated. I measured his pulse and oxygen levels every five to ten minutes, performed suction every two hours in order to clear his breathing pathways, and fed him the food he could digest, as well as foods we were hoping he would be able to digest.

In the little time we had left during the day, I would sing to him, play with him, try to make him laugh, and inspire him to move through various games and activities.

After a few weeks, I reached out to find someone that specialized in teaching toddlers to move. While researching the Feldenkrais method, I stumbled upon the *Tzaad Rishon* method, meaning "first step" in Hebrew. I signed up, and over the course of six months, the trainers of the program worked with Arieldavid and taught us innovative ways to help him learn to move. After a few weeks, I began to better understand my son's external and internal worlds as I witnessed the immense impact of movement on his breathing, his vital energy, and his happiness.

Our living room became a playground filled with physical therapy equipment, as well as Pilates balls, books, musical instruments, and more. I tried almost everything to encourage Arieldavid to move without forcing it on him. Here, creativity and my background as a children's exhibition designer came to my aid. I noticed that laughing and playing music motivated Arieldavid to move! Thank God, he moved! I was so proud of him. Despite all he had gone through, he chose to follow the music and move. He chose, by himself, without words, to put the pain aside for a few moments in order to move. He was and still is my role model in happiness and good nature. Slowly, day by day, his condition improved.

One month after we arrived home, the chief nurse came to visit us with the chief doctor of the children's ICU. They were incredibly happy to see that Arieldavid was doing fine. Just before they left, the doctor told me that he did not think we would survive even one week at home. I thanked him for not sharing this with me at the hospital before we were discharged because I was so hopeful and eager to help my son live a happy life at home that I only needed words of encouragement and not doubt or disbelief. Overall, I was extremely glad to hear the doctor say it because, for me, it was a sign that maybe we were doing something right; maybe we were on the right path after all.

When the weather was nice, Arieldavid's breathing was stable, and I had the courage to take him outside for a walk, I would put him in a double stroller with all the medical equipment that he had. I laid him on one side of the stroller, and the ventilation machine, suction machine, a five-liter oxygen tank, and an oxygen level monitor on the other side. With a baby bag on my back, filled with food, diapers and an Ambu device for manual ventilation, we headed up the steep streets of the Carmel Mountain in Haifa.

Arieldavid loved going outside. Our walks took us as far as the neighborhood playground and back home. We could not stay out for very long because he required constant medical treatment, and his medical equipment required electricity. This was incredibly stressful for me as I was constantly alert and anxious, but seeing the smile on my son's face made it all worth it. Such a small thing as a one-hour walk outside was a huge victory for us. It was uplifting and gave us enough strength to make it through the day, move forward, and not be overwhelmed with stress and anxiety. Coping with stress was one of the main issues I faced as a mom to a child with a life-threatening health challenge. I realized I needed to learn how to soothe myself in order to be available for him, to tend to his needs and to help him live a full and happy life without imposing my fears and worries on him.

We had very few visitors, and our days were very busy from morning till night. There were, however, a few people who did come over regularly and had a substantial and positive impact on our life. Two of them were my mother and her partner, who, with their sunny nature, spread a lot of light and happiness around us. My mother had to adjust to all the medical equipment, which, for her, was not an easy task, as she always said, "I'm just not a technical person." Yet, in her special way, she became extremely involved with Arieldavid and his progress. There was deep love between the three of them, and I felt blessed to see this. I loved my son so deeply and was happy to see him loved by others as well.

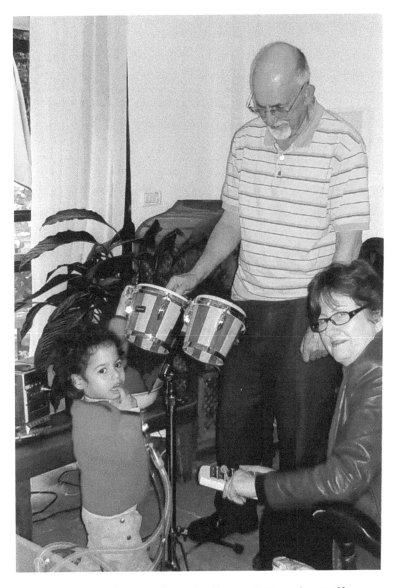

Arieldavid, Grandma Atalia, and Grandpa Jeff,
playing music together, 2011

Another weekly visitor was Sveta, who was an educator for toddlers with special needs. She was working in Peuton Hashachar, managed today by Elvin Israel, and decided that if Arieldavid could not come to kindergarten, she would bring the kindergarten to him. For six months, Sveta volunteered to come every morning for thirty minutes before going to the kindergarten where she worked.

Sveta played with, talked, and sang to Arieldavid, and he loved it! One might think that thirty minutes is not a lot, but for Arieldavid, it was a whole new beautiful world. It diverted his attention from the monitoring, check-ups, and medical treatments.

I learned a lot from Sveta and continued to do what she showed me after she had left. I felt blessed that a complete stranger went out of her own way to help make our day brighter. I felt humbled to witness such kindness from a fellow human being.

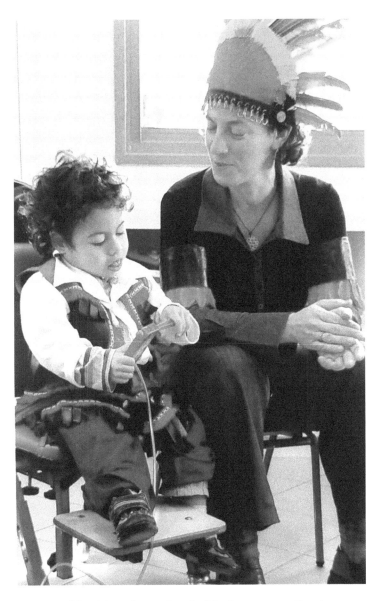

Arieldavid and Yamina in kindergarten: Peuton
Hashachar, Purim Party, 2009

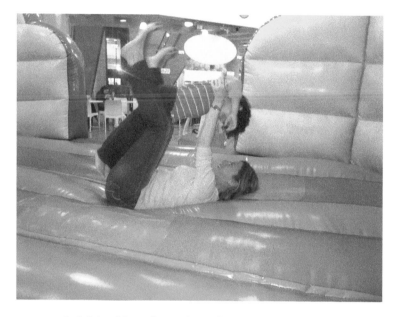

Arieldavid and Yamina playing at Jamboree
Playground, 2011

The Lightworkers of This World

Throughout the day, there were unexpected medical emergency situations that resulted in me needing to ventilate Arieldavid manually, using the Ambu device, which is an external airbag that connects to the ventilated person and pumps air into the lungs via a squeezing motion. This must be done in a very relaxed manner, with full concentration on the person being ventilated so as to avoid harming him or her. Incorrect use of the Ambu may create excessive air pressure that might cause the lungs to burst and lead to death.

This devastating event is exactly what happened to Arieldavid when he was in the hospital at the age of one month—a nurse used the Ambu in a way that caused my son's lungs to blow up, causing him to stop breathing altogether. It took twenty-one minutes to bring him back to life, and he was never the same afterward. During those twenty-one minutes, no oxygen reached his brain; this most likely caused the long-term cognitive damage that is apparent to this day.

Having gone through such a horrid, painful event, I felt very cautious and anxious when using the Ambu. It was an extremely dangerous procedure that left my body in a state of stress way after Arieldavid was breathing normally again. There were days when I had to use the Ambu on Arieldavid around thirty times to help him breathe. During these times that he stopped breathing, he began to spasm, and his body became hard and blue. This condition, in which children stop breathing and faint, is called a "breath-holding spell."

Normally when a child has a breath-holding spell, loss of consciousness brings back the breathing, but in Arieldavid's case, the breathing depended on the ventilation machine, which was not suited for such extreme situations, and so manual interventions with the Ambu device were necessary to keep his oxygen levels stable. These spells continued for about five years. As a result, our life became very intense physically, mentally, and emotionally.

There was hardly any balance in my or my son's life. I did not even know where we would find ourselves at the end of the day—at home or in the hospital's ICU and for how long we would remain there. Each morning at dawn, I thanked God for letting us pass another night and live to see another day. As dramatic as it may sound, it was actually far more dramatic. And this dramatic life started to take its toll on my health and emotional capacity.

I became very irritable. I felt that my adrenaline level was running high almost twenty-four hours a day. I hardly slept a single night without waking up in a panic to ventilate my son with an Ambu when he stopped breathing, and during the day, I monitored and performed medical procedures on him. I also tried my very best to play with him and encourage his curiosity to learn and to explore the world around him, to make him laugh and feel happy. There was no option for me to even go to the toilet, shower, or eat properly as he had to be watched over all the time, in sleep and in waking hours as well. My every basic need was rushed, if at all acknowledged. It was extremely difficult to live like that, and I knew that my body and soul were paying a heavy price.

My mother pleaded that I make some changes. She was afraid that this stressful life would kill me. "I have to protect my son," I told her. "I have no other choice but to live this way."

Little did I know that a few lightworkers were already on their way to help us.

One day my mom called me and said, "A good friend of mine, Adam, wants to meet you and Arieldavid. He wants to help."

"What can he do?" I asked my mom with little faith.

"Let's find out," she said. "Adam is a remarkable person and likes helping people," she added.

Back in the day, my mother and Adam Fish had worked together in the human rights movement. They had stayed in touch, and when he heard about Arieldavid, he offered to help.

When Adam came to our house, I thought that he was very warm and friendly and a keen observer. He quickly understood our situation. He asked me many questions regarding Arieldavid's medical status: what kind of support was our health insurance providing? What did our daily routine look like? And what would we need to live a balanced life?

I gladly answered all his questions. I felt heard, and that gave me relief. I shared with him my frustration that in order for my son to live, I had to sacrifice my own life. I said I barely slept, ate, or worked during the days when I watched over him.

At the end of the meeting, Adam said, "I'll help you get what you need for Arieldavid to live at home, and you will get to live as well."

I did not really believe him. I thought he was just being nice. But a few days later, I got a call from Moshe Fibich, who was working with Adam and Rachel Ben Ari in their law firm, and he invited me to come in the next day for our first official meeting.

For the next six years, Adam Fish, Rachel Ben Ari, Professor Moshe Fibich, and the Haim Cohen Justice Center for the Legal Protection of Human Rights fought in court for Arieldavid's rights to receive the necessary medical equipment, a medical caregiver, and special paramedical treatments at home, such as physical therapy, speech therapy, and occupational therapy. They made four appeals to the district court and one appeal to the supreme court. They won all the appeals.

It was a miracle that changed our lives forever. It enabled us to provide Arieldavid with the help he needed, as well as begin to return to our own lives as people. They put hundreds of hours of work into these court appeals, and they asked for nothing in return; it was all good will, pro bono.

One day, after six years, we were getting ready for our final court appeal, and I was exhausted. Adam turned to me and said, "Your son is my good luck charm." I was so moved when I heard that. He did not pity us; he had tremendous respect for our daily efforts. "Don't give up," he added, "You are a hero; things will work out. It takes time to change the system, but once you take one block out of that huge wall, it all comes down. This is what we are doing: we are taking down the wall."

He was right. Things did take a long time, but we did succeed. Adam, Moshe, and Rachel were our angels who did the impossible to help Arieldavid receive his rights to live like any child. No words can truly express how grateful I am to them.

A few months after we won our case, Adam unexpectedly died. It was shocking to grasp that he was really gone. Yet his legacy, and what he believed in, lives on in my son and me, as well as in the many lives of other families who began to receive benefits thanks to his efforts.

The results of the court appeal that Adam, Moshe, and Rachel conducted echoed for many years after they finished, as it also impacted the lives of others with similar life circumstances. This was achieved by the efforts of the welfare office that was managed under the care of social worker Gadi Pollack, who was the principal manager for the north district. Gadi Pollack was an extraordinary man who never stopped thinking about what else he could do to assist others like us. It was thanks to his efforts that children like Arieldavid, who were living at home and could not go to the kindergarten, received assistance and educational treatments at home.

We also learned that after all the appeals we had done, the awareness for ventilated children grew, and there was a higher budget allocated to their needs by their health insurance. Of course, this could be a coincidence or a ripple effect, but whatever the cause, I was happy things began to shift for the better for people that were suffering from things similar to what we were going through.

We tried to convince the Ministry of Health to create a budget for ventilated children that would protect their rights to live at home and receive adductive medical and educational assistance. However, we were not able to make this change a reality.

All this made me realize how important the efforts of individual people can be. We don't have to simply rely on politicians and hope for the better; we can also push the envelope ourselves with whatever skills and authority we have at the moment, trying to make a positive difference in the lives of others. It was thanks to these kinds of people that Arieldavid and I were able to transform our lives. It took a long time, but after all these years, I could finally start to focus some of the time on my own health and well-being as well.

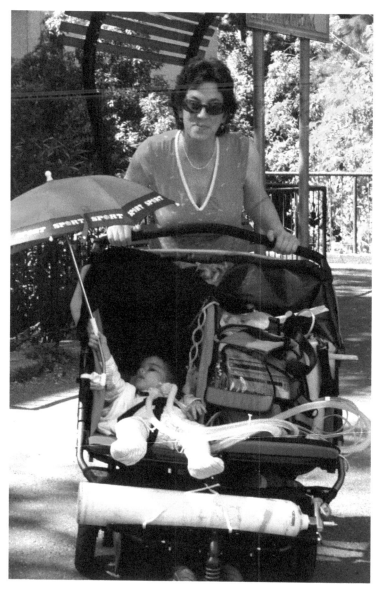

Arieldavid and Yamina with a Tween stroller and
ventilation machine, 2006

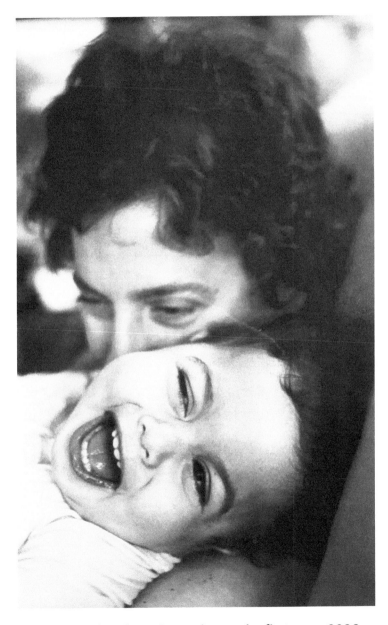

Arieldavid and Yamina at home the first year, 2006

The Tree Meditation

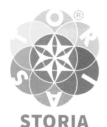

STORIA

Overview: We all have moments when we find ourselves lost in the deep woods, not knowing which direction to go. We feel anxious, frustrated, angry, depressed, and helpless. This is a good moment to stop, sit down, and dive deep inside ourselves. When we are at peace, the mind is still and clear, and the light can shine through and show us the way home.

Preparation

Sit on a chair with your two feet on the floor or on a pillow with your legs crossed. Find a comfortable position while making sure you are sitting upright with your back straight. Put your hands on your lap and slowly close your eyes. Inhale through your nose and slowly exhale through your mouth.

Steps

1. See the tree

   Imagine you are standing in an open field of grass. At the center of the field you see a single immense and extraordinary oak tree. Get closer to it. Look at the trunk of the tree and notice how stable it is. Reach out and touch the tree. Feel its royal presence. Now gently hug the tree; lean on it completely, and feel its texture against your cheek.

2. Release all worries

Now you can really let go. Just melt into it and listen to its sounds. Let go of all the thoughts and worries that trouble you. Let all the stress come out of your body through your head, up into the branches, and into the leaves of the tree. And as the wind blows, hear the rustling sound of the leaves releasing all these tensions into the air. See the sunshine through them as they dissolve in the atmosphere.

3. Reveal your core value

- **Enter the intimate space**: Now bring your attention back to the trunk of the tree and begin to breathe with it. Inhale through the nose and slowly exhale through the mouth. Feel the tree's slow and rhythmic breath. Notice the heartbeat of the tree and notice how strong and steady it is. Effortlessly allow yourself to blend and merge with this rhythm. Let yourself dive deep into a peaceful internal space where you and the tree can have an intimate conversation.

- **Ask and receive**: Feel the tree's heart open as it reveals its warm and inviting essence to you. You get the feeling that you are in the presence of an old friend that you have known all your life. Now open your heart and greet him while letting him know that you appreciate his loving presence. Now that you are reunited, kindly ask him to remind you what your core value in life is. Listen to the answer closely, and feel it in your heart as the words become clearer and clearer. Do not change anything. Openly receive any image, thought, feeling, or emotion that arrives. Give in completely, and let the truth of who you really are be revealed in this sacred space. Let the value of your soul be spoken, and let it connect you to your higher self, which is longing to live this life passionately from within the core value.

- **Be grateful**: Thank the tree, and let it know how much you appreciate the gifts that it shared. Know that your souls are now connected, and you can always come back and talk to the tree in this deep and intimate space that you created together. Sanctify it, and in return, the tree will always give you love and honest answers that resonate with your higher self.

Conclusion

Take a deep breath. As you exhale, slowly open your eyes.

If you wish, contemplate on the value and/or the image which appeared. Ask yourself how you can create this image and value in your life. What conditions would you need to create in your life in order to manifest this value? What specifically would you need in order to make these conditions possible in a gradual and harmonious way?

The man who at will can assume whatever state he pleases has found the keys to the Kingdom of Heaven. The Keys are desire, imagination and a steadily focused attention on the feeling of the wish fulfilled. To such a man any undesirable objective fact is no longer a reality and the ardent wish no longer a dream.

–The Power of Awareness *by Neville*

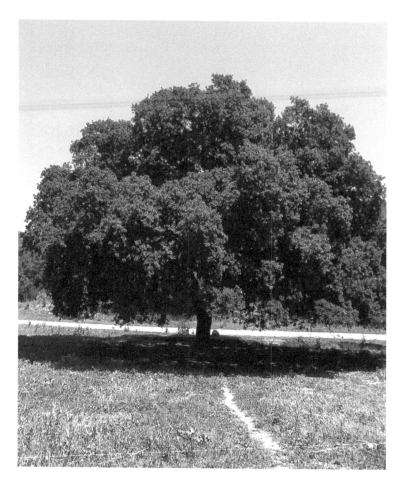

Big, beautiful old oak tree, 2021

CHAPTER 2

Saint Francis and the School of Self-Awareness

A very important moment in the work on oneself is when a man begins to distinguish between his personality and his essence. A man's real I, his individuality, can grow only from his essence. It can be said that a man's individuality is his essence, grown up, mature. But in order to enable essence to grow up, it is first of all necessary to weaken the constant pressure of personality upon it, because the obstacles to the growth of essence are contained in personality.

**– In Search of the Miraculous:
Fragments of an Unknown Teaching**
by P. D. Ouspensky

A Day of Joy Before the Storm

By the end of the first year of Arieldavid's life, there was no trace of my previous life. My marriage had ended. My career was about to end, and my financial means were almost exhausted. Most of my friends and relatives were nowhere to be found. I felt that I had become a shadow. The only light that kept me going was the love for my son and the hope of healing him while giving him a chance to live a full and happy life.

It was the beginning of the winter of 2006. Arieldavid had just turned one, and we were celebrating his birthday party at home. It was a rare, joyous day. After everything we had gone through, we were finally celebrating. Friends, family members, and people I had not seen in a very long time came to our home. It was a nice change, and I felt very grateful. I realized that for many of them, seeing us go through such a hard year was not easy, and the disappointment and hurt I felt from them transformed that day into gratitude. The fact that they came to my son's birthday celebration, accepting him as he was, was a big gesture for many of them.

It was a moving event. The garden was full of children, laughter, and pure happiness. There was music in the background as the guests offered their blessings, wishing Arieldavid and me a happy life. My heart was filled with gratitude for this wonderful day.

The next days were spent in pure joy. We were beginning to come to terms with the rhythm of our daily life. As hard as it was, there was peace in finding some stability in the unstable circumstances of our life.

In *Yoga Sutras of Patanjali*, in Chapter 2, the sutra *Sthira Sukham Asanam* means: "Yoga pose is a steady and comfortable position." This sentence can refer not only to the yoga postures, but also to our daily lives, beyond the yoga mat. This quote from Patanjali made me think about my own life and ask myself, "Do I have balance in my life? Am I comfortable and stable while facing daily challenges? How do I react to challenges? How are my body, mind, and spirit affected by the challenges I face?"

I felt that I had coped with my challenges in the best way I could up to this point, but still I was wondering, "Could I do this better?" If the idea of a stable position in yoga could be projected into daily life, it meant that the challenges I was facing didn't need to have a stressful effect on me, which they did. "Is this possible?" I asked myself again and again. The more I contemplated these questions, the more I noticed how much stress was cooped up in my body.

During these days, it felt like we finally reached a stable rhythm in our daily life. However, those few days of happiness were cut short and without warning as I found myself holding Arieldavid in my arms while being rushed in an ambulance to the intensive care unit at the Children's Hospital in Rambam. I felt as if death had arrived at our doorstep and was hovering over Arieldavid.

In the hospital, they were barely able to stabilize my son's condition. The doctors explained that he had an intussusception in the intestines. This is a serious condition of the inversion of one portion of the intestine within another, causing a bowel obstruction, blocking food and fluid from passing through, which can lead to death within a very short time.

The next months were spent in an ongoing battle between life and death. After three surgeries, a solution was still nowhere to be found. All efforts were futile. It felt like every time we tried to swim toward the shore, we were thrown back into deep waters. We were struggling to keep our heads above water while gasping for some air before making another attempt to reach a safe harbor.

I felt hopeless, devastated, and unable to move. I had never felt this way before. There were always new ways, new solutions, but this time, I could see none. These thoughts and emotions of helplessness pushed me deep inside myself, urging me to find a solution and look at my situation from a different perspective. This was my first real attempt to be in *Svadyaya*, self-study. From that point on, this term became more than just a word, but a path I attempt to walk on.

The Book, the Bookmark, and the Quote

There is a life form found in the deepest and darkest place on earth. In the depths of the ocean, where hardly any life exists, where there is no light, you can find beautiful, self-sustaining, glorious, luminous living creatures that illuminate the darkness with their light. The time in the hospital, for me, was a time in which darkness was all around me, and there was no light to be found. I needed to reach into the depths of my own soul to find my light. I needed to shine it so strongly and so brightly that someone in the universe could see it and come to my aid in rescuing my son.

One day, while I was sitting by my son's hospital bed, a visitor came in and handed me a gift, saying, "I was standing in the bookstore downstairs, looking for a book to read, when I saw this book. I thought it would be perfect for you."

I thanked him for his thoughtfulness, as I was reading many books during my hours there. I looked at the book and read its title out loud while contemplating the words I was pronouncing: *In Search of the Miraculous: Fragments of an Unknown Teaching.*

What does it mean? I asked myself. Inside the book I found a bookmark with a quote printed on it. The quote read: *There is no place where you can be free; there is only your place. Only there can you find freedom. –Patrizio Paoletti.*

I didn't know who Patrizio Paoletti was, nor did I know Ouspensky, the author of the book. I did, however, know a bit about Gurdjieff, whose ideas were presented in the book. A few years earlier, while still living in New York, I had come across some of Gurdjieff's ideas and books. A good friend of mine attended a group inspired by Gurdjieff's ideas and told me about the changes she had experienced as a result of studying these ideas.

The quote by Mr. Paoletti resonated with me deeply. To be able to save my son against all odds. Against all the medical statistics and advice. Against all the heartbreak I was going through. Against all the pain I witnessed my son tormented by. Against losing my own identity as a wife, as a friend, and as a careerwoman. Against all that, being able to sustain my own solid choice of sanctifying my son's life and actually being able to create the life I was visualizing. For me, this meant freedom.

"What if it's true? What if you can live out your inner vision? Not only dream about it, but actually do it. But how can it be possible when you dream of the impossible? What would I need for this to happen? What would I need to change in my son's life or in my own?"

These questions ran through my mind as I wondered who could teach me how to do this.

The other side of the bookmark contained a school's name and a phone number. It read: "The School for Self-Awareness for the Harmonious Development of Man." It was in that moment that I knew the universe was responding to my prayers.

Deep in my heart I knew that the book, the bookmark, and the quote on it were not a mere coincidence. I had already seen enough to know that there was a thread of energy that connected my life's story with something bigger than myself. I knew intuitively that there were "lightworkers" sensing that I was looking for help, telling me, "Yes, this is possible. Go on. Continue. Do not be afraid. Do not give up. Stay strong. You are not alone. Help is on the way. You're on the right path!"

In the next few days, my mind was busy planning my next steps. I remember thinking that once I get Arieldavid out of the hospital, I could join the school and meet Mr. Patrizio Paoletti. I believed that as a founder of the School of Self-Awareness, he must have deep and vast knowledge about the human mind and body. And so, upon meeting him, I planned to ask him how I could teach my son to breathe by himself. I decided to take a leap of faith and join this school. But first I needed to get my son back home.

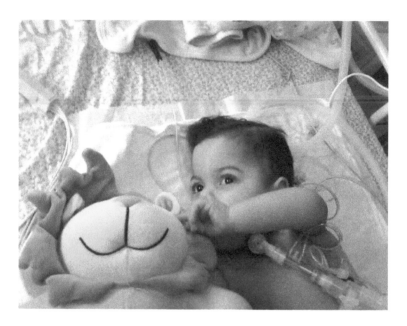

Arieldavid in the ICU, 2006

The School of Self Awareness for the Harmonious Development of Man

After four months in the hospital, Arieldavid's condition was stable again and we were able to return home, thank God! The decision I made at the hospital to join the school was firm. I called the number on the bookmark upon our arrival back home. A few days later, I met two students from the school in a coffee shop. They came to interview me. They told me about the nature of the School of Self-Awareness, the rationale behind it, and its goal: the evolution of mankind. This evolution is only possible when man becomes aware of himself and changes his nature, which can be achieved by work in a group directed by a teacher who has completed the path himself.

To me, it sounded like a very meaningful goal, but it held little interest for me, as I had my own personal goal in mind: to find a way to heal my son. And though I was curious about the possibility of evolving to a higher state of conciousness and being, I felt it would be very selfish to focus my attention on anything but helping my son to heal.

I made my goal clear to the students and hoped that I could make use of what I was about to learn at the school to achieve my personal goal. They praised me for having a personal goal because they said it could be a source of power, especially in times when energy was lacking. They called these periods of time "an interval in the octave" and explained that to get out of these intervals, a "shock" is needed to help you remain on the path toward the goal you initially chose. So your goal can be used as fuel for the fire that is burning in the engine that drives you forward.

Within a short time after that meeting, I was notified there was one more interview that had to take place before I could join the group meetings. I was told that Mr. Paoletti had received the information about me and would soon decide if I might be accepted into the school.

On the night before meeting the facilitator of the Haifa group for this last interview, I had a dream. I dreamt I was in a small room with twenty-four pillows, twelve on the left side and twelve on the right. There was a large candle at the front of the room, with stained glass windows behind it. I felt relaxed and at peace.

I then entered a different room and met Patrizio Paoletti, who greeted me with a warm smile. I woke up and knew that I was accepted into the school. This "knowing" was based on an intuition that was like nothing I had experienced before. I was curious to understand what kind of dream it was, and I wanted to learn this ability that enabled one to reach places while in a state of sleep.

Sure enough, I went to the interview, and a few days later I was notified that I had been accepted to the school and was welcome to attend group meetings in Haifa. One month after entering the school, I was already on my way to Assisi for a school retreat in Le Case, hoping to meet with the teacher, Mr. Paoletti. There, I hoped to receive an answer to my question on how to teach my son to breathe independently.

When I arrived at Le Case, I felt a need to pray and asked the facilitator of the retreat to enter the little chapel. When I entered, I was filled with peace. The light was dim; only one candle lit up the place. When my eyes got used to the darkness, I could look around; to my surprise, the place seemed to be very similar to the one from my dream.

Saint Francis and the Power of Visualization

The Creative Power within us makes us into the image of that to which we give our attention.

–The Science of Getting Rich *by Wallace D. Wattles*

I arrived in Assisi in the early hours of the morning. The retreat was scheduled to begin on the next day in the afternoon at Le Case, which was located an approximate forty-minute drive into the mountains of Umbria, just above this ancient Middle Ages city.

There was a full day at my disposal, so I decided to make my way up to the famous church of Saint Francis, "La Basilica di San Francesco." At that time, I had no knowledge of who Saint Francis was, but all of Assisi was dedicated to this man, with images of him in every shop. Besides, realizing how preoccupied I was with the question I wished to ask Mr. Paoletti, a stroll to the church seemed like a pleasant diversion that would ease my mind a bit.

As I began to walk through the streets of Assisi, I felt my heart beating very strongly. I thought to myself, *It's not only my mind that needs relief but also my heart that is carrying so much pain. I feel it might burst.*

As I walked, I noticed that I was repeatedly chanting, "Please help my son be healed. Please show me how to help him to be healed." In my mind, I kept seeing an image of my son in his early teens, healed and happy, with his beautiful smile. I had seen this image in my mind during my time at the hospital by my son's bedside. This image was like a lighthouse showing me which direction to take on a dark, stormy night. This image had brought me here, to Assisi, in the most unexpected way.

After some time, I reached the entrance to the church. Having a prayer in my heart and the image of my son healed and happy in my mind, I entered the church. It was the entrance to the upper level, where, I later learned, there were original, six-hundred-year-old huge wall paintings (frescos) by Giotto depicting the life of Saint Francis of Assisi. As I mentioned before, at that time I did not know about Saint Francis or about Giotto.

I paced slowly from one wall painting to the next with wonder. I was drawn to one fresco painting in particular. It had the figure of Saint Francis with direct lines connecting his hands and feet to another figure in the sky. It was, as I later researched in the church's bookshop, the painting of the stigmata of Saint Francis, where, as legend has it, Saint Francis was so absorbed by his devotion to Christ that he became like the crucified Christ, bearing his wounds.

As I observed the painting attentively, I noticed Saint Francis's facial expression intensely focused upon the crucified figure above, his body seemingly free of all tension. There were lines connecting Christ's wounds to the same places on St. Francis's body. I was stunned. *Here is my answer!* I thought to myself, barely able to stop myself from shouting out loud, *Eureka!*

I was born and raised in a Jewish home and had no direct contact with Christianity, except for when I was growing up in London and went to public school with children with diverse ethnic and religious backgrounds. I know my excitement was not based on religion, but solely on this extraordinary human experience.

Even if the stigmata did not really happen, I thought, *it is a beautiful legend that tells the tale of an extraordinary Transformation with a capital T.*

For me, this story was inspirational beyond words. The idea that eight hundred years ago this man focused his mind, his deeds, and his words solely on becoming someone else, with such intensity to a point that his body transformed to accommodate his vision, was absolutely awe inspiring. This was an amazing act of manifestation through imagination. The act of seeing clearly in advance the desired future while taking the necessary steps in order to reach it. Realizing this, I thought, *This is a great sign for me that I am going in the right direction.*

It *is* possible to do the impossible. I just needed to know the steps I had to follow to reach the future I saw for my son and I would do it! If only I had some kind of a magical map to show me the way.

Through observing the painting, it seemed that the answer was right in front of me: "All you need to do is see in your mind's eye what you want to become and go in that direction." It was amazing! It was exactly what I had been doing with my son by holding the image of him happy and healed. I was astonished by this realization and by the fact that someone else had embodied this idea eight hundred years ago. This made me think that there was much more to our potential abilities than I had previously thought possible.

I kept thinking to myself, *How is it possible that we are not taught how to imagine the future from an early age in kindergarten and school? It is our birthright. How wonderful would it be if we had this knowledge? If only this knowledge was taught and practiced, it would change the approach of hospitals to the management and healing of diseases. It would reduce stress and suffering and give strength, resilience, and hope to countless people.*

In that moment, in the church, looking at the wall painting, my magical map of how to reach my vision was still very far away from me. I left the church and headed back to the hotel. The next day I traveled to Le Case with great hopes of meeting Mr. Paoletti.

The Retreat

The Meaning of Life, I doubt whether a doctor can answer this question in general terms. For the meaning of life differs from man to man, from day to day and from hour to hour. What matters, therefore, is not the meaning of life in general but rather the specific meaning of a person's life at a given moment. To put the question in general terms would be comparable to the question posed to a chess champion: "Tell me, Master, what is the best move in the world?" There simply is no such thing as the best or even a good move apart from a particular situation in a game and the particular personality of one's opponent. The same holds for human existence. One should not search for an abstract meaning of life. Everyone has his own specific vocation or mission in life to carry out a concrete assignment which demands fulfillment. Therein he cannot be replaced, nor can his life be repeated. Thus, everyone's task is as unique as is his specific opportunity to implement it. As each situation in life represents a challenge to man and presents a problem for him to solve, the question of the meaning of life may actually be reversed. Ultimately, man should not ask what the meaning of his life is, but rather he must recognize that it is he who is asked. In a word, each man is questioned by life; and he can only answer to life by answering for his own life; to life he can only respond by being responsible.

–Man's Search for Meaning *by Viktor E. Frankl*

The morning of the retreat had finally arrived, and the excitement began to flow in my veins. At the hotel, I asked the concierge at the front desk to call the taxi I had booked to take me up to Le Case. I wanted to leave earlier than planned so I might have some time to stroll around before the retreat began.

The taxi came, and as we began our ride up the mountains of Umbria, I noticed how magical this place was. We drove along a beautiful, curving road. I could see Assisi in the distance, as the taxi turned onto a small side road leading into deep woods. The car window was open, and a current of fresh air washed in. I could smell the leaves and the trees.

This brought up a distant memory of a part of my childhood spent with my family in England. The nature there had a positive impression on me. I loved being surrounded by nature; it always had a calming effect on me and made me joyful and lively. The scenery was reviving and uplifting. Up until that moment, I had forgotten how much I needed nature around me. I had always known this in the back of my mind, but had never taken it as an essential part of the life I wanted to have. I noted to myself that I should take this into account when I got back home.

When we reached Le Case, a peaceful feeling came over me. There was peace in this place, which I so dearly needed. I noticed a few aesthetic stone houses that had been built in an orderly fashion. I entered one of the buildings to register. It was a harmonious space, with just practical furniture. I registered and received the schedule for the retreat. The place was also very organized and clearly charted. It seemed that there were no accidents in the design in the entire place, as if each brick and plant had been carefully choreographed to generate a specific feeling: peace. For a few minutes I spontaneously entered into a thought-free state of stillness.

The retreat began in the afternoon. The hall was packed with people, and we received a very tight schedule of practices. It started at seven thirty in the morning and ended around eleven thirty at night. There was a time scheduled for meditation, eating, working, studying, and special movement sessions. These movements were called sacred movements and quickly became my favorite part of the day. I got most of the movements wrong, but they astonished and excited me. I was intrigued and wanted to study these movements. Oddly enough, even when I got the movements wrong, I was not at all preoccupied by it. Just seeing them performed by the facilitator brought inexplicable joy to my heart and peace to my mind. As I continued, I could sense my mind entering a harmonious state.

Sometimes One Question Requires Much Planning and Practice

At the beginning of the retreat, I asked Mr. Paoletti's secretary whether I could meet with him, but she could not give me a definite answer. I stayed hopeful that an opportunity would present itself and every day tried to prepare myself for asking Mr. Paoletti my question. On the first day of the retreat, I had the good fortune of meeting a very special woman named Padide with whom I felt a natural connection. As soon as I shared the reason for my coming to the retreat, she suggested I practice how I would ask Mr. Paoletti the question. *How hard could that be?* I thought.

But apparently, even one question requires a lot of planning and practice. When you have so little time to talk with someone, you must be very accurate and clear about what you are asking. You need to be aware of your true motivation for asking and about how you expect the answer to affect you.

On the third day of the retreat, I still had not received an answer from Mr. Paoletti's secretary regarding the possibility of meeting him. It was not yet clear whether he was coming to the retreat at all. "But either way," I said to myself, "Be ready to ask the question as if he was definitely going to meet you, and leave the rest to God's grace."

I trained as hard as I could to be completely prepared in formulating the question, as well as balancing my emotional state. I was so emotionally involved with my son that merely thinking of his current condition brought tears to my eyes. I really had to pull myself together in order to ask this question. I needed to speak from a place of detachment that would allow me to remain calm and not burst into tears while talking about my deep yearning for my son to live and be healed.

The Teacher and the Question

The days went by, and I still could not get an answer as to whether Mr. Paoletti would meet with me. I had traveled far for this opportunity to meet him and was not ready to leave without getting an answer. I felt like a lioness trying to protect her cub and who would allow nothing to prevent her from doing so. Of course, there was one thing that could prevent it—time and the airplane I needed to be on to get back to my son.

Even a lioness has limits, I thought. The retreat was almost over, and I was coming to terms with the fact that I might not achieve my goal. But just as I was ready to give up on asking my question, it was announced that Mr. Paoletti had arrived unexpectedly to give the retreat participants a short teaching.

There was a lot of excitement in the air. People were rushing from one building to another, tidying up and bringing chairs into the large hall. Several hours later, we all sat in anticipation as Mr. Paoletti came in. The hall became silent, and everyone stood up. He walked to the front of the hall. His walk was brisk and elegant, and he gave the impression of stability while at the same time almost hovering above the ground. He seemed to be dancing in space. I felt that he was with us completely, and at the same time, almost in another world. He was like no other man I had ever met before.

He sat down in front of us and asked us to sit as well. I was very nervous and alert. I knew exactly what I would say to him if the opportunity presented itself as I had been practicing with Padide every day. Now, thanks to her help, I was ready to do my part. *This is my only opportunity to ask him my question,* I thought, *but how should I do it? I can't just interrupt the teaching.*

The teaching was about to begin, and I thought I would have a couple of hours to find the right moment. But to my surprise, Mr. Paoletti looked at us, and as if he could read my mind, he asked, "Who here has a question for me?"

He is talking to me, I thought. *Wake up! And raise your hand fast!* I swiftly raised my hand to receive the microphone.

I never anticipated that my opportunity to talk with Mr. Paoletti would include a few dozen people. Suddenly, the realization that I was about to speak about a private matter in front of all these strangers reached me, and for a few long seconds, I found myself unable to move or breathe. I felt self-conscious in the audience's presence as I perceived myself as a shy person. Having Padide at my side gave me strength, and I reminded myself why I was there.

I kept thinking of my son, and by the time I received the microphone, my fear was gone. "*Shalom*, Mr. Paoletti," I greeted him in Hebrew. "I'm a mother from Israel, and my son is now one year old. He was born without the automatic breathing command. And as a result, he has been ventilated from birth. I came all the way here to ask you if you could guide me in how to teach my son to breathe independently."

I asked my question and looked straight at Mr. Paoletti, waiting for his answer. I was somewhat calm and focused. I had attained my goal and asked him my question, and now I was waiting for the result without any expectations, only with the hope that there would be something I could do to help my child heal, something I could chart on my magical map.

The hall was completely silent. I did not even want to look at the audience because I knew they were probably in shock, and I was afraid I would start to cry.

Then Mr. Paoletti said, "This is a very big subject, and I will talk with you personally later."

He then went into a deep teaching about motherhood and the role of a mother. He gave the example of Mary, mother of Jesus, and how she willingly and actively played a role in protecting the life that was bestowed into her hands. Later, I would study her story deeply as I found her to be very inspirational; a story about a mother's unconditional love for her child and about unconditionally trusting in God.

Padide turned to me and whispered, "He is answering you. Can you see that?"

Mr. Paoletti was saying things that, at that time, I did not understand. *How is this connected to me and to my life?* I thought, *And when will he talk with me? The retreat is ending tomorrow.*

The Teacher and the Answer

The next day, we reached the end of the retreat, and soon after lunch, I got ready to go to Rome, where I was going to catch a plane back home. I thought that Mr. Paoletti would probably not come as he still hadn't come to talk to me. I was eating lunch quietly with my head bent. I felt empty and did not really know what my next step ought to be. I felt I had reached a dead end.

Suddenly, the door to the dining room opened, and everyone became silent at once. *Mr. Paoletti certainly knows how to make an entrance*, I thought, and felt as though his arrival revived my hopes.

"Dov'è la ragazza Israeliana?" he asked, surprising me. I realized he was looking for me. I immediately jumped out of my seat and walked over to meet him. With one simple gesture, Mr. Paoletti invited me to exit the dining room.

I followed Mr. Paoletti around the stone building, and he pointed to some chairs overlooking the garden and the mountain view. *What a beautiful landscape*, I thought.

For the next hour, Mr. Paoletti and I talked about Arieldavid's health condition and the ways I might be able to assist him. I shared with him my vision for my son to be able to breathe independently and live a full, healthy, and happy life. He listened to me without judging me. I felt his compassion;

it felt as if he was listening directly to my heart. He was not trying to shut me up with statistics and the lack of possibility of this happening.

Mr. Paoletti did not give me direct instructions but rather offered me some options and directions for me to consider and research. He did not talk with me directly about breathing techniques, but rather about the conditions that would stimulate my son's cognitive ability and communication through play and other methods.

At the end of our meeting, I told him that whatever he would give me through his teachings, I would pass on to my son, and later on, with God's grace, to others as well. I was happy to have had this opportunity to talk to him and was completely grateful for his genuine approach to me and my story. *What a great man!* I thought. *Despite his immense responsibilities and his very busy schedule, he still manages to make time and attentively listen to the people that he doesn't even know and give them advice from his vast knowledge.*

Over the next six years, almost every time I met Mr. Paoletti, he would hear about my son's progress and give me his advice. But to me, more than anything else, Paoletti was a symbol of hope. He truly believed in mankind. He believed that man could change and evolve, and that gave me a lot of hope for my own quest to evolve and help my son heal.

Mr. Paoletti's teachings reflected his belief in the best version of oneself, one's highest potential as a human being, and the possibility of each man to reach it.

To me, Mr. Paoletti was the air that I needed to breathe in order to have the strength to go on until the reality I envisioned came true. He was the bridge between my external reality and my internal vision. His words and recommendations opened new worlds for me.

One of these worlds was "*guarire.*" A year after I met Mr. Paoletti, I received the amazing opportunity to learn how to be a vessel for the light. *Guarire*, which is the Italian word for healing, is the application of healing energy through the practitioner. In *guarire*, practitioners put their hands on various locations of the participant's body in order to transfer the cosmic healing energy of God's grace that is around us and in us to the individual receiving the *guarire*.

I practiced the *guarire* technique on a daily basis with Arieldavid for over four years, and to this day, we practice it three times a week. Through this practice, Mr. Paoletti helped me realize that we are so much more than we think we are, and there is so much parents can do to help their children at any given moment. The practice of *guarire* made me feel like an active participant and not just a bystander in my son's healing. It also allowed me to realize the interconnection we all have with each other in a spiritual yet practical way. It helped me to reconnect with a higher level of consciousness that supports my son and me, and all of us, in fact. And it helped me realize that there are things beyond my comprehension, but this does not prevent me from participating in the beautiful, all-inclusive dance of life. For me, this was a humbling realization.

For this reason, when the practice of *guarire* begins, the practitioner always begins by saying, "It is not I, but rather it is you that is here for me." With this saying, the practitioner declares that he is aware that there are greater forces at work, and he is only a channel and not the source of energy that is being transferred to the participant.

Arieldavid's condition was improving day by day. His life was sustained many times thanks to *guarire* and thanks to many practitioners that I had no contact with directly, but I received the information that my son was being cared for by them with *guarire* healing energy sent to him from afar. Knowing this was reassuring, especially during the traumatic emergencies that we still faced. For me, *guarire* was an active form of praying, which helped me take more responsibility and be more involved in my son's healing. It gave me purpose and hope. It was uplifting and life-sustaining, which, for me, meant keeping my world intact.

Paoletti's teachings of self-awareness enabled me to distinguish between imagination and reality. Thus, in crucial moments when despair crept in, I remembered my goal and was able to overcome it, moving forward toward a full and happy life for my son and, eventually, for me as well. The answer Mr. Paoletti gave me at the retreat was, in fact, received with time through the practice of self-awareness. The answer was not one thing that I could do, but rather a series of conditions I would need to create around my son, as well as in my internal and external world, so his natural healing process could occur in an organic way.

The role that Mr. Paoletti and the School of Self-Awareness for the Harmonious Development of Man played in my life was both spiritual and practical. There are not enough words to describe the importance of having a mentor that believes in you and in what you do. I felt that Mr. Paoletti believed in me as I believed in my own son. For me, this was a core source of power, which gave me enough strength to go in search of a miracle to reach my goal to heal Arieldavid and free him from the ventilation machine.

The teachings and exercises I received in the school were the vehicles with which my knowledge of how to reach my goal was gradually attained. This knowledge is not transferred through books, though there are books in which these ideas are presented. But rather, this knowledge is gained through individual efforts, practices, self-observation, meditation, and contemplation on our human experience and the effects of the world around us.

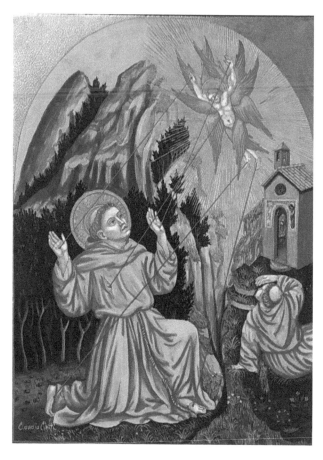

An interpretation of Saint Francis receiving the stigmata, commissioned by Yamina for Arieldavid's third birthday as a reference for him and her to visualize the healthy, full life they both wish for. Painted as interpreted by Claudia Ciotti. The original is a fresco from the thirteenth century, attributed to Giotto Di Bodone, located in the Basilica Di San Francesco, Assisi, Italy, 2008

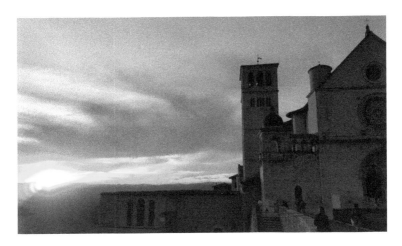

Basilica Di San Francesco, Assisi, Italy, 2017

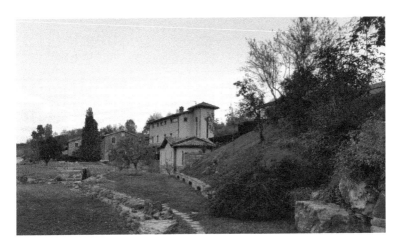

Le Case, near Assisi, Italy, 2017

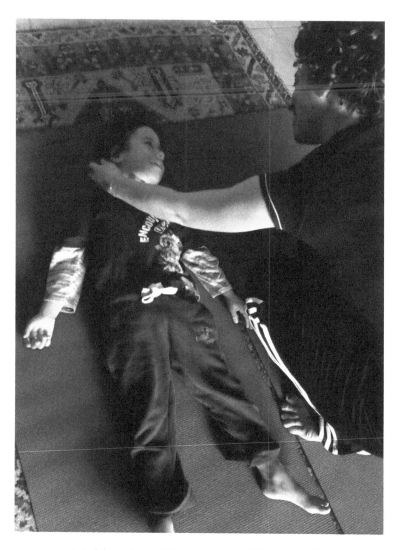

Arieldavid and Yamina practicing guarire,
healing energy, 2010

The Rock Meditation

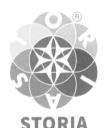

STORIA

Overview: This is a short meditation I experienced spontaneously while my son was in the ICU during one of his longest hospitalizations. One day, after sitting by his side for many hours while he was sleeping, I decided to get some fresh air and went out of the hospital for a short stroll. The children's hospital was right near the sea, so I walked to the rocky shore and sat down on one of the rocks. As I was gazing into the sea, I noticed a large rock in the distance that peeked out of the water as the waves washed over it.

I looked at this phenomenon for a good few minutes and began to feel a relaxed sensation in my mind. It was as if all my worries were washed away with the water covering the rock and then left to shine in the sun. The rock remained solid and stable, even though it seemed to be in the most unsuitable, unstable, unforgiving place; it made it very clear to the surroundings that it was not moving anywhere. This was very symbolic to me. I felt identified with the rock as I, too, remained firmly established in my core value— to cherish my son's life, helping him fulfill his potential, regardless of the circumstances.

Consistent efforts in the direction of one's core value require both faith, determination, and detachment from the end result. In other words, whatever happens, you keep on going. "Until when?" you may ask. Until you have succeeded in manifesting your inner truth into the world. Of course, this does not mean at any cost. No, it means that with a balanced attitude, you find a way to do just the next step on the path you chose. And then another one, and so on. The rock meditation will help you maintain a firm direction on your path.

I wish you the best of luck in using this meditation as your personal anchor for firmly holding your core value, your truth, your aspiration.

Preparation

Set the place for your meditation. Take time to prepare it, as this is a sacred place.

The place should be clean and quiet. You may also want to light a small candle and incense (sandalwood is always recommended). Turn off your phone and other electronic devices for the next fifteen minutes as you invest this time in yourself. Sit comfortably in an upright position on a yoga mat, a pillow, or a chair. Close your eyes softly, inhale deeply through your nose, and slowly exhale through your mouth. Relax yourself more and more with every breath you take, feeling the weight of your own body as your awareness expands in all directions, beyond your body's outline.

Steps

1. The rock is stable

   Take another deep breath and imagine you are standing on the shore looking into the ocean. In the distance you can see a marvelous rock peeking from the water like a lotus flower. You see how huge waves crash on the rock again and again, but it remains strong, firmly grounded and completely unmovable. See yourself sitting on this rock. Take a good look at it and see it in detail. Really examine it. Smell it. Feel its texture. Feel its unyielding stability, its unchanging permanence.

2. The rock is alive

   Remember your core value and breathe it into the rock; see the rock light up in a beautiful golden color and come to life. This rock is your core value, and the waves are all of your life's challenges and instabilities, all of your worries and fears that strike you again and again. Hug your rock and know with all your heart that as long as you are here, you are safe, and no wave can wash you away. Notice how the waves around you begin to disperse and quiet down as they see that they are no match for your rock. The sun comes out from behind the clouds, and you notice birds flying and dolphins swimming around you, jumping high and diving deep.

3. The rock nourishes

The water is now still and clear; you can see far into the depths of the ocean, and you realize that this rock is immense! Far bigger than you imagined! In fact, it's not really a rock, but more of an island, spreading wide and deep, reaching the bottom of the ocean. When you look closer, you can see life all around the rock, above and below it. Birds, sea turtles, corals, plants, fish, and other creatures that live in a harmonious ecosystem, all nourished by your island. When you live from your core value, when you hold onto it and try to manifest it into the world, you not only nourish yourself; you give life to everything around you. Ask yourself now: How does your core value bring life into the world? How does it nourish the people around you—your husband or wife, your kids, friends, parents, your neighbors, and your community?

Conclusion

Now that you have recharged your faith in yourself and in your truth, you are ready to return. Take a deep breath and very slowly and calmly open your eyes. Don't move your body for a few seconds. Let yourself get used to the surroundings before you engage with it. Slowly move your body and come back fully to the here and now.

Know that you can always return to your island any time you feel insecure about something, are worried, fearful, or have doubts and anxiety. This meditation will help you regain your inner strength to continue on your path.

.

CHAPTER 3
The Magical Map

That person, who always eats wholesome food,
enjoys a regular lifestyle, remains unattached to the
objects of the senses, gives and forgives, loves truth,
and serves others, is without disease.

— Vagbhata Sutrasthana

How Can I Strengthen Arieldavid's Body, Mind, and Spirit?

From the very beginning of Arieldavid's life, his breathing and digestive system were the sources of our challenges. From birth, his physical health was unstable. He was connected to the ventilation machine all the time, and the bowel obstruction was still a source of much suffering.

I constantly faced the question of how I could strengthen Arieldavid's body, mind, and spirit. In the dream I had on the night he was born, my reply to the man standing in our hallway was, "How? I know all will be okay, but how? What am I to do?"

For many years, the "how" question motivated me to look for solutions through research, study, trials, and observations. At times, I didn't know where to look for solutions, and sometimes the solutions seemed bizarre and impractical, but I didn't give up and let my intuition guide me. Some of the paths I chose didn't always make sense to the mind; however, they made perfect sense to my heart. I realized that I had no real frame of reference as my son's condition was very rare. I decided to break down the "how" question into smaller subjects in order to understand exactly what was needed for my son to heal and develop.

I was overwhelmed by the many things I had to research and learn in order to help him. It seemed it might require the work of a lifetime to create the conditions for his healing to occur. And I would have to do all of this in parallel to monitoring him, managing his medical state, his breathing and the function of his digestive system, as well as promoting his cognitive development, while working to make a living and looking after a household, and of course, trying to find time to just be a mom. As you can imagine, this was not an easy realization for me. It meant that it was not a sprint but rather a lifelong marathon in which Arieldavid and I were the sole runners.

But the second I thought of the love for my son and his happiness when his life would be full and healthy, I was able to put aside my own fears and frustrations and chart a list of the specific conditions to improve our situation. But it was more than just a list, more of a road map, and so I called it my "Storia Map," since it was the map that helped me navigate my life and gave me a chance to rewrite my life story and create the story that I actually wanted to experience. The story where my son has the perfect conditions to heal and live a full and happy life with me.

The first version of the Storia Map was in the form of a list of possible beneficial conditions and approaches, which then were sorted into categories. With time, the Storia Map evolved into a method with a deep and detailed representation of the possible courses of action to reach one's deepest aspirations. Today, the Storia Map consists of imagery, key words, and other methods to help clearly visualize the life story we wish to manifest.

Note: In the last chapter of this book, I will share with you how I built the full Storia Map for Arieldavid and explain how you can build your own Storia Map.

After outlining the categories, I divided each section into subsections and then converted each category into a daily/weekly/monthly/yearly outline of goals. At that time I couldn't imagine that in the future, Arieldavid would develop hobbies such as wall climbing, horseback riding, and even bicycling. But I could imagine the outline of the conditions needed for such a full life to be manifested.

Since Arieldavid was a baby when I began to compose this list, I had to step into his baby shoes and try to understand what he might need in order to purify and strengthen his body, mind, and spirit. I came up with the following sections, knowing that, with time, as Arieldavid became more independent, he would modify this list to suit his personal needs and preferences. Each section stands alone, but they work together holistically, affecting one another.

- **Breathing**
    - Free of external invasive ventilation
    - Free of external monitoring
- **Movement**
    - Movement indoors
    - Movement outdoors, especially in nature
- **The interior surroundings of our home**
    - Loving
    - Warm
    - Safe
    - Peaceful
    - Quiet
    - Positive
    - Relaxed
    - Aesthetic

- ❏ Organized
- ❏ Clean
- ❏ Uncluttered
- ❏ Full of light

- **Fasting**
  - ❏ Emergency fasting with vein infusion at the ICU when signs of life-threatening conditions arise due to constipation
  - ❏ Fasting at home with vein infusion in the initial stages of constipation to prevent escalation and hospitalization
  - ❏ Preventative intermediate fasting during seasonal changes and/or the beginning of a cold

- **Nutrition**
  - ❏ Digestible medical and nutritional supplements
  - ❏ Natural ingredients: mainly fruits and vegetables
  - ❏ Very small portions of organic dairy products like smooth cheese or ghee
  - ❏ Vegetable and chicken soup with small portions of organic chicken
  - ❏ Organic eggs two to three times a week

- **Emotional Well-Being**
    - Laughter and happiness
    - Social engagement and companionship
    - Interests and hobbies
- **Cognitive Skills**
    - Language and communication: vocal, sign language, and computer-aided
    - Games
    - Reading
    - Writing
    - Math
    - Art
- **Hobbies**
    - Things Arieldavid would love to do
- **Life Skills**
    - Independence
- **Guardianship**
    - Someone who would watch over him and his interests when I am old and unable to do so myself.

This list allowed me to see the bigger picture and plan ahead the small details of how, where, when, and what conditions

I needed to create, including the people and knowledge I would need to access for this purpose. After planning all this, I researched each category and met the people who were experts in that area to discuss how it could be adapted to improve my son's condition. Then I introduced it to my son in a fun way. If he liked it, we continued, but if he or his body declined it, we would adjust the approach or stop and move to another option. This, in a nutshell, was the whole process from A to Z.

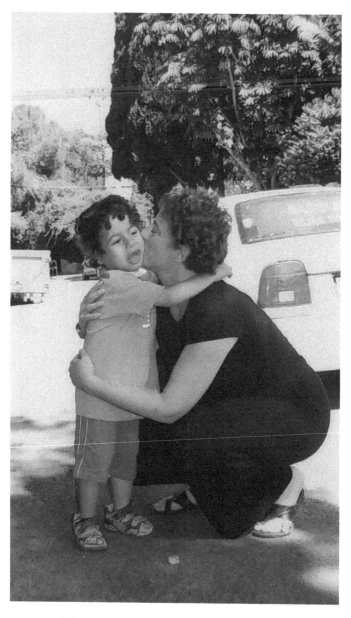

Arieldavid and Yamina having a stroll, 2009

From Outline to Reality

You'll see it when you believe it.

–Wayne Dyer

Breathing and Movement

The Storia Map was the outline for giving answers to the "how" question. But from the outline to actually getting results, well, that was an entirely different story. And the best place to start, I thought, was looking at what was most urgent. This was, of course, Arieldavid's breathing and the reoccurring constipation of his digestive system.

I started to look for answers while still in the hospital. When I held my baby boy and put him over me, I would talk to him softly. Sometimes I would just hold him quietly while listening to his heart beating. His tiny body would relax in my hug. Both of us would enter another world, even if for a short time, and the world would consist of happiness and peace. These moments were immensely valuable for my son and me.

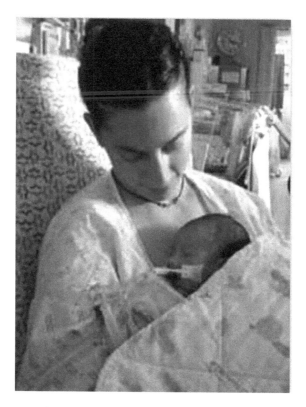

Yamina holding Arieldavid, skin to skin, a few days after Arieldavid's birth, ICU, 2005

After Arieldavid was born, while at the hospital, with the medical staff standing by, we would try to disconnect Arieldavid from the ventilation machine almost every day but with no success. One day, one of the doctors came up with another suggestion. He said there was a researcher that claimed that the breathing system may be activated through movement. The research suggested that ventilated patients showed signs of independent breathing when their foot was constantly moved during sleep. The researchers actually designed a machine that would move the foot all night.

So, as funny as it might sound, it was far better than seeing my son ventilated twenty-four-seven. You can probably imagine what I started doing for many hours. But even then, the movement of my son's tiny baby foot did not induce independent breathing. Time passed, and there was no improvement; he remained ventilated at all times.

During that period, my son went through much physical and emotional suffering, which left him very weak and traumatized. I realized the most important thing would be to get him home, and only there would we start our path toward healing again. I was very grateful to the doctors and medical staff who saved his life and enabled me to take him home at the age of four months old.

After spending so much time in the hospital, returning home was a blessing that allowed me to shower Arieldavid with warmth and love. However, soon after we arrived, it became apparent that the apartment we lived in was not suitable for a ventilated baby. It was on the third floor and made it very hard for me to bring in all the medical equipment; I had to go back and forth to the car, which made it very difficult to monitor Arieldavid's breathing. It was nearly impossible unless there were always two people, but this was not really a realistic option. It became very apparent—we had to move.

Luckily, after a short period of time, we found a house that was perfect. It was on the first floor and was easily accessible. It had a huge living room, which became Arieldavid's playground, in which we spent most of our waking hours. There were big floor-to-ceiling windows overlooking the vast sky and the trees in the garden. It was beautiful and peaceful, and I thought it would be very good for my son to grow up in this house.

After we settled in, we returned to our Storia Map outline. Breathing and movement were our first concerns. We continued to try different ways to motivate Arieldavid to move. It became very clear how breathing and movement are strongly connected, affecting one another. When we move, our breathing becomes deeper and more frequent, oxygenating the mind and body, activating our digestion system, and helping with waste elimination and absorption, which in turn helps us to be more active.

One day, about a year later, I entered my son's room, and he was lying on his back in his crib with his head bent backward; his back was arched while his chest was open and directed to the ceiling. To my surprise, he was very relaxed and content. It looked like a yoga posture I had seen once.

I later read about this posture and learned its name in Sanskrit, "*Matsyasana*," the fish pose. Among other benefits, with practice, this posture helps to improve breathing. I was very excited to see that Arieldavid's body was intuitively trying to help itself and decided it would be beneficial to study more body movements that could help him. Through my studies and my own observations of my son's healing process, I began to realize that the body has inner wisdom and naturally tries to balance itself under the right conditions. This was strongly linked to my basic intuition that God helps us work out whatever obstacles we undergo.

God always leads us to find a doorway and a key that will open it; all we have to do is search for it. My intuition kept telling me that somewhere there had to be a key that would open the internal healing power that my son naturally possessed. From what I saw that day, it was a clear sign that the key to substantially improving his breathing was yoga.

A few weeks later, I began to study integrated yoga with Zipi Negev at her course in Ramat Hasharon. This was an advanced course that certified yoga teachers. Luckily, Zipi was very understanding and open to the fact that I had no prior background in yoga, and she constantly said, "What you are doing with your son is yoga." At that time, I did not understand what she meant. It took me over a decade of studying yoga to understand that yogis are not just the ones who know the body postures (asanas), but also the ones who dedicate their lives to improving themselves and others by following the path of yoga—the path toward unity, self-awareness, and self-healing.

In the book *Gheranda Samhita – Commentary on Yoga*, Swami Niranjanananda Saraswati writes, "A common definition of Yoga is union between the individual consciousness and the cosmic consciousness." This is a four-stage process. First, the person is a seeker (*jignasu*), then a devotee (*sadhaka*), then one who has attained truth and knowledge (*yogi*), and lastly, a liberated soul (*jivanmukta*).

Studying yoga enabled me to practice movements with my son that were suitable for his needs and abilities. In time, the world of yoga opened up something deep within me as well. I was able to connect to my own spiritual path toward truth and unity, which I had long neglected even before my son's birth. And it is thanks to my son that, with time, I learned to be devoted to this path and to see how it was improving my own well-being, my motherhood, and ultimately affecting how I worked with people, assisting them with their own growth.

For my son, the yoga mat was the first place where he changed from being dependent to becoming independent. The two of us have been practicing yoga together for over ten years now. It has given Arieldavid strength, confidence, joy, and, more importantly, a sense of autonomy and the ability to move and to breathe independently.

In yoga, even when there is an intent to reach a state of consciousness or a body posture, there shouldn't be expectations to reach that goal. The practice is done with a pure heart and dedication, which in time creates a path for the movement of vital energy to go through the entire body. One can think of this as the unfolding of a blooming flower, which adds a beautiful range of colors to life itself. As a mother of a ventilated child, yoga has been the place where I witnessed my son change, becoming more independent both in body and in spirit. Even when he was still ventilated, in the first years of his life, there was so much power in him, just sitting gracefully in a perfect *Padmasana* (lotus pose).

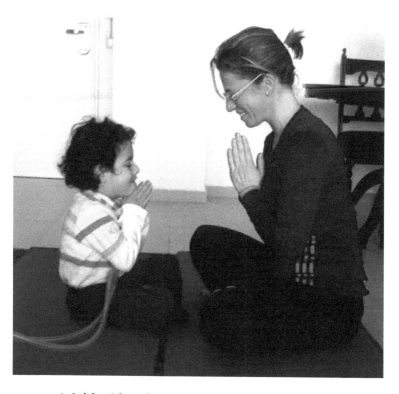

Arieldavid and Yamina practicing yoga, 2014

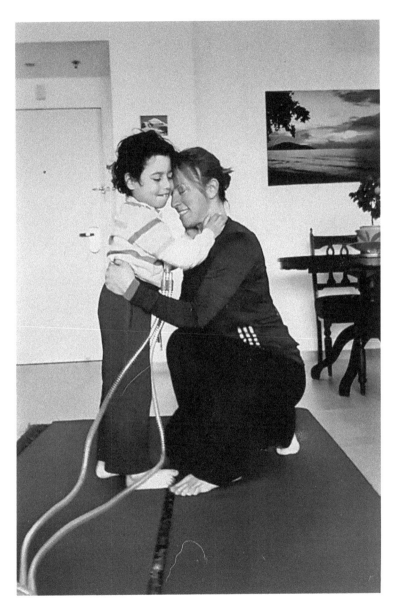

Arieldavid and Yamina practicing yoga, 2014

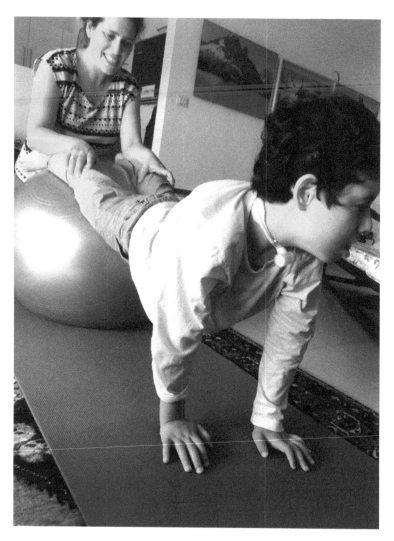

Arieldavid and physical therapist Naama Yaari, 2015

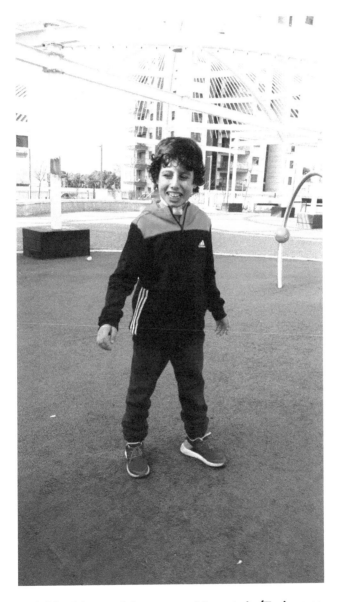

Arieldavid practicing yoga, Mountain/Tadasana
Posture, 2016

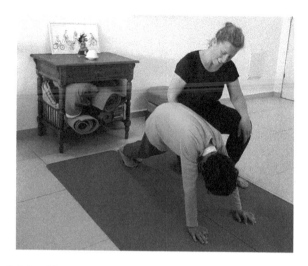

Arieldavid practicing yoga, Downward-Facing Dog/
Adho Mukha Svanasana Posture, 2017

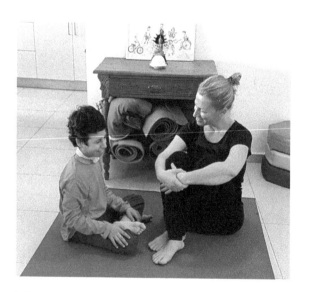

Arieldavid and Yamina practicing yoga together:
Easy Sitting/Sukhasana Posture, 2017

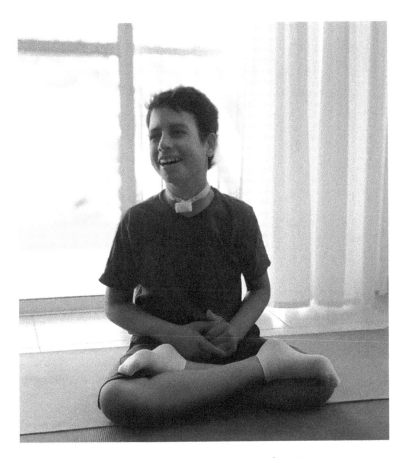

Arieldavid practicing yoga: Lotus/Padmasana
Posture, 2020

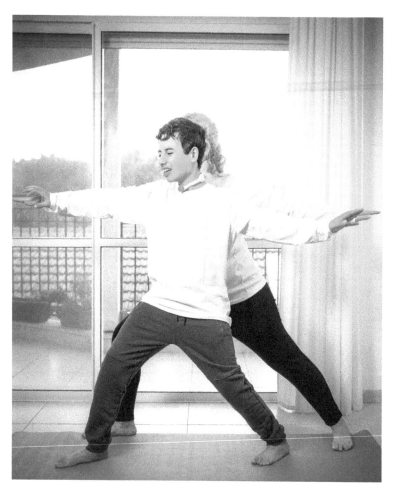

Arieldavid and Yamina practicing yoga: Warrior/
Virabhadrasana II Posture, 2020

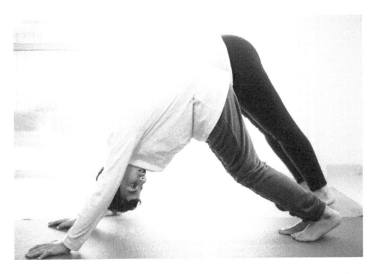

Arieldavid and Yamina practicing yoga: Downward-Facing Dog/Adho Mukha Svanasana *Posture, 2020*

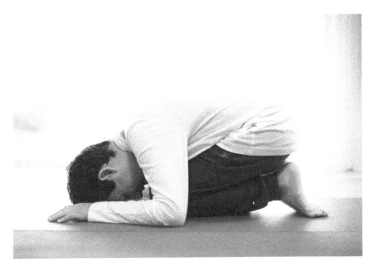

Arieldavid practicing yoga: Child's/Balasana Posture, 2020

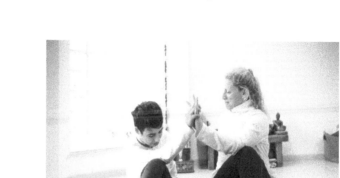

Arieldavid and Yamina practicing yoga: Seated
Twist/Marichyasana III Posture, 2020

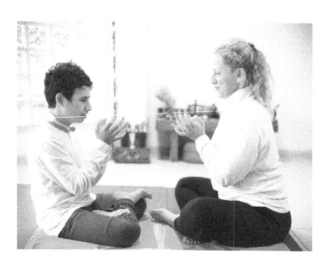

Arieldavid and Yamina practicing Bhrigu *yoga:*
Lotus/Ambuj Mudra Exercise, 2020

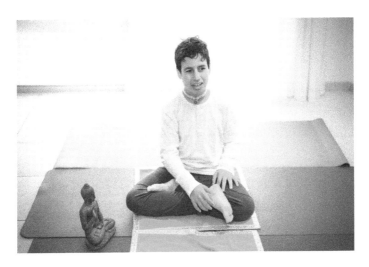

Arieldavid practicing yoga: Lotus/Padmasana Posture, 2020

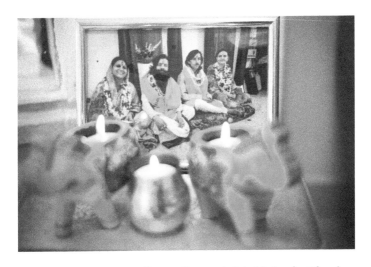

Homage area to my Guru. From right: Vatsala Bhadury, Dr. Jayant K. Bhadury, Acharya Hemant K. Bhadury and Mithlesh Kishori Bhadury, 2020

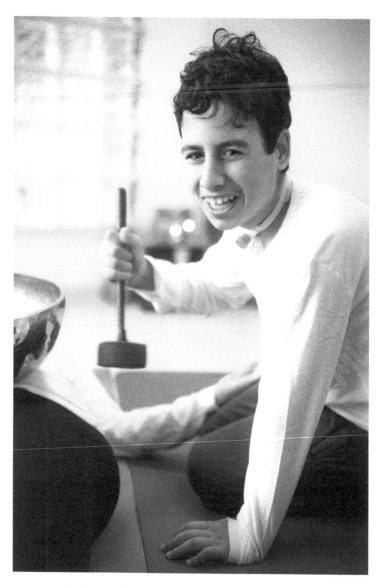

Arieldavid and Yamina practicing rejuvenation with
Tibetan Singing Bowls, 2020

Fasting and Nutrition

In the early years of Arieldavid's life, food, the digestion of food, and the elimination of waste was an extremely big issue that many times resulted in the need for fasting.

Hirschsprung disease, which was the second obstacle for his health, kept pulling us five steps back each time we managed to move one step forward. Because of Hirschsprung disease, Arieldavid's digestive system was not functioning properly from the day he was born. Even after nine surgeries, we were still facing severe problems that brought us to the ICU to endure long periods of fasting, time and time again.

"What can I do? And where can I learn to do it?" I asked myself these questions so many times. But, unable to reach any other solution besides going back to the ICU in the hospital, I turned to my mother for advice on alternative medicine, with which she had some experience. My mother suggested that I meet with Pnina Bar Sela, who was a well-known expert in cleansing and rejuvenating the body and the digestive system through fasting and healthy eating habits.

Arieldavid was one year old when I met Pnina at her home in Kiryat Tiv'on. I asked her bluntly whether he could fast at home.

"Fasting?" Pnina repeated, her face revealing how terrifying the thought of a one-year-old toddler fasting was to her. "Only adults can and should fast. And they, too, need, in some cases, medical supervision," she replied.

I nodded, knowing that it was true, as I had seen how the hospital's medical staff was very cautious with Arieldavid's fasting. Yet this question came as a result of my deep need to free my son from the traumatic effects of hospitalizations and find, in a loving and warm environment, a way to solve the constipation he went through at home.

What will I do now? I thought to myself, horrified by the idea that we would have to stay dependent on the hospital. Everything I was trying to build would be threatened if we had to return to the hospital again and again. All the hours I spent trying to uplift my son's spirit would be lost during the emergency drives to the hospital. There was nothing I could do except witness the destruction of our efforts, over and over again, trying to rebuild Arieldavid's faith in life from scratch every time we returned home. The agony and pain we both associated with the hospital were so severe that they pushed us to work really hard and with dedication to improve his strength and health while at home.

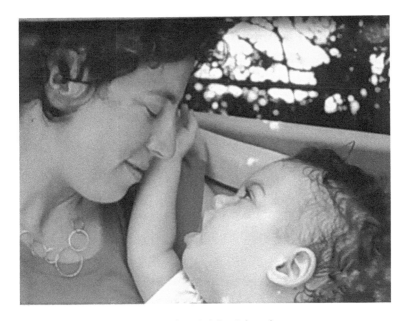

Yamina and Arieldavid at home,
AD a few months old, 2006

Frustrated by the fact that my son's life was again in the hands of the hospital, I felt helpless. There was nothing I could do but pray and wait until he was older. But waiting is not easy when a loved one is in much pain and suffering. Regardless of my sleep deprivation, even when I had the time, it was very difficult for me to fall asleep. Even on quiet days, I was worried that any day the next attack might happen, and my son would be rushed to the hospital. No, I could not just sit and wait—so I didn't. I searched and searched for solutions.

A few years had passed. My son was already three years old and still in and out of the hospital every few weeks because of severe constipation. There they treated him with monitored fasting and several additional operations on his colon, but sadly there were still no enduring results.

My mother then suggested that I go to Mitzpe Alummot Health Farm, which at that time was run by the founders and owners, Jerry and Edna Mintz. They were kind to us and let us stay in a beautiful apartment. However, Arieldavid was not able to participate in all of the activities of their thoughtful health program as he was still very young. I did, however, learn of the importance of a healthy daily routine that included practicing breathing through movement, walking in nature, and having healthy green juices and shakes. At home, I tried to offer my son juices, but they were not well received by his body, and once more, I needed to wait for a while and try again.

When Arieldavid turned eight, I still intuitively believed that fasting at home would be more beneficial and therapeutic for him than fasting in the hospital, which could expose him to viruses and diseases, as well as trigger pain-related memories. At that age, Arieldavid was already showing signs of post-traumatic stress syndrome in hospital settings. He had shown signs as a toddler as well, but at the age of eight, on top of the physical pain of constipation, his emotional suffering became even more apparent when entering a hospital.

On one occasion, when my son was beginning to show signs of constipation, I could not bear the thought of taking him to the hospital and seeing the traumatic effects again. I decided, *It's enough; there has to be another way.* I telephoned his family doctor and pleaded to be allowed to try to help my son at home by performing a fast that we would monitor carefully and thoughtfully, starting with some water and sugar and seeing how that affected his digestive system. Of course, if there were any signs of distress, I would immediately rush to the hospital. Being very humane, and aware of Arieldavid's traumatic suffering and the dangers of exposure to bacteria in the hospital, especially for a ventilated child, the doctor agreed.

Arieldavid was relieved to do this at home. He fully cooperated, knowing that it was better than being in the ICU. Most of the time, drinking water with sugar was sufficient and produced the desired results. However, on a few other, more severe occasions, his doctor had to intervene and perform a vein infusion to provide my son's body with water and sugar, letting his digestive system rest completely from anything entering through the mouth.

Fasting at home was peaceful, and we were able to assist Arieldavid anytime he needed help. The constipation would be relieved, usually between twenty-four to forty-eight hours of fasting, without needing to go to the ICU. We only needed to return there again once.

One day Arieldavid was very sick when he returned from school and required immediate medical assistance. We rushed him to the emergency room, where he was treated and discharged after four days. Besides this one episode, we learned to read the physical signs before the problem arose and acted in accordance with the body's needs. Luckily, as Arieldavid grew and became stronger, he stopped suffering from constipation altogether, and fasting was no longer needed. This, of course, was an immense blessing for his health, growth, and happiness.

At some point, when Arieldavid was about seven years old, after learning about all the benefits of fasting, I, too, began fasting once a week, which I still do today. The fast is called "The 16 Monday Fast" or "*Somvar Vrat.*" In India, this one-day fast, once a week, over sixteen weeks, is seen as a practice that will help you attain anything you wish for. Once again, patience was a core theme in my life, as I wished for big things many years ahead.

I found that fasting works powerfully on a spiritual as well as on a physical level. On the physical level, I feel that fasting rejuvenates the life force within me as it cleanses my digestive system that affects my whole body, including the mind. On a spiritual level, I often feel more available to go deep into contemplation on why I am here, from my role as a mother, a wife, a yoga teacher, and a meditation instructor, but also, and perhaps more importantly, on my role as a fellow human being.

For many years we continued trying to give Arieldavid fruit shakes and juices, and thank God, at the age of fourteen, he was able to finally digest fruit juices and fruit shakes like his favorite banana and apple shake with almonds and dates, which he loves to drink and helps to prepare himself! Seeing how much Arieldavid enjoys his morning routine and food in general is yet another example that it is worthwhile to try and try again, even if it takes years to find a suitable solution in order to witness the desired results.

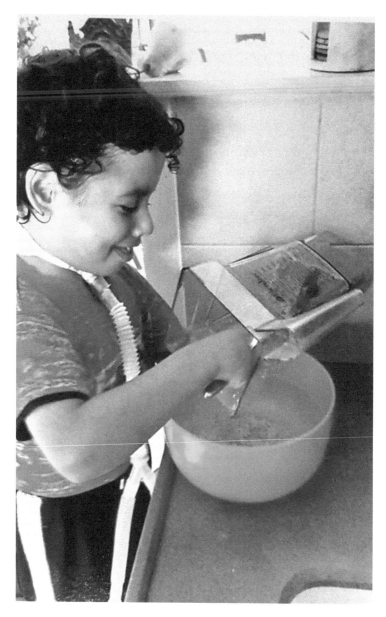

Arieldavid assisting in preparing food, 2012

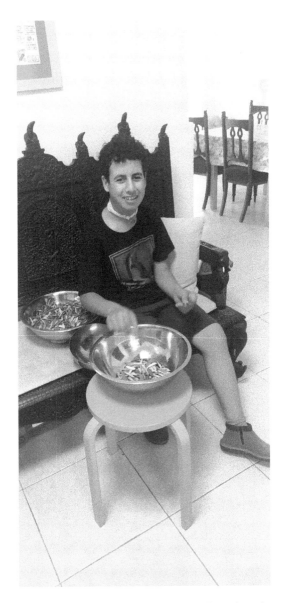

*Arieldavid Assisting In preparing the olive leaves
for infusion, 2021*

The term "to wait" or to develop patience is well rooted in the fundamental concepts and practice of yoga. Every step in yoga is developed slowly and with sincere practice. After a period of time, you wake up one day and, just like a flower that has blossomed overnight, you find that the practice has changed you. Your body and mind have changed for the better, and you can use the benefits you have attained through the practice to bring them to your daily life, to your loved ones, and to your community. All this is based on continuous practice, which requires steady patience and constant endurance to keep trying without expectation or judgment of the result. Without this process, which I learned through studying and practicing yoga and meditation, I would not have attained anything I so wished for.

It is in this section that I wish to also share with you an exercise I developed as part of the Storia Map to help me better understand what I wanted, needed, and could do in order to improve my son's life, as well as my own life. I call it "My Life's Exhibition Exercise." I use the realizations from the exercise to know what seeds are needed in order to obtain the fruits in my and my son's life. I invite you to try it, too, to find the seeds you want to plant in order to manifest the story you want to live.

My Life's Exhibition Exercise

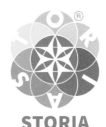

STORIA

Overview: The purpose of this exercise is to remember and review the most significant moments in your life in order to understand your core value. These meaningful moments hold a strong emotional charge within them, which affects our thoughts and beliefs and therefore our actions and behavior. If we choose the right moments and analyze them sincerely, they will become a reliable mirror that will clearly show us our true selves as we were, as we are, and as we might become. If we look closely, this mirror will reveal our core values—our true motives and desires, our true purpose in life. And once you know your purpose, you will stop wasting your time and energy on peripheral needs and begin to redirect your precious resources to attain what truly matters. I wish you the best of luck in finding your core self, as it will benefit you in many ways and fill you with happiness and peace.

This exercise is about creating a review of highly significant moments in your life. Try to identify the core life value you were manifesting in your actions and trace back the origin of that value. When in life did you obtain this value, and why?

Who contributed to this? It may be that you witnessed a negative experience or a negative action by someone else, and this contributed to the development of this value in you. Or it may be that you witnessed someone behaving so benevolently toward you that you wanted to behave in the same way toward others. Alternatively, it may be your own value, born out of your core or your yearning to behave in a specific way that you believe is the right way for you. Whatever the origin of your value is, the important thing to emphasize is how this value empowered and motivated you to make the changes within yourself in order to act in the way that brought the achievements and goals you had at that time.

Understanding how your value directed your thoughts and, therefore, your actions in a certain way will help you to use this knowledge for the second step of this exercise, which is to predict your own life's exhibition twenty-five years from now, as well as the values you will need in order to get there. This second part will also be the foundation for "the Farmer's Meditation," where you will use this information to choose which value seeds to plant today in order to grow the fruits you wish to harvest in the future. I wish you the best of luck in finding your core self, as it will benefit you in many ways and give you happiness and peace.

The Goal

The goal of this exercise is for you to observe that you are already a winner and that you have already achieved many things in your life. It is important, before going out into the world with a new life mission, to see what strengths you already possess within yourself and to learn how you obtained them and what influenced you. This exercise will also help you to orient your life twenty-five years ahead and to see where you want to be then as you look back to this day. This will help you to assess what values are required in order to reach those future results and to direct your thoughts and actions accordingly.

Preparation

Arrange to have some uninterrupted quiet time for yourself.

Step 1

Try to recollect the seven most meaningful events, which you feel best represent who you are and what you believe in.

Then, for each of the seven events, write:

- What was the event?
- Why was it meaningful to you?
- What values did you express in this event?

Step 2

Go over the seven events you have listed. Try to see them as one big picture—your self-portrait. What do these events have in common? What do these values have in common? Try to extract the underlying key value, which encompasses within itself all the other values.

Conclusion

These are deep and important questions, and it might take a long time to receive a clear, satisfying answer. So, if you are still not clear on what your core value is, don't give up; repeating this exercise will help you to refine your answer and turn your beautiful light into a powerful laser beam that can permeate through any obstacle.

Nevertheless, if you made a real effort, I'm sure that by now you at least have a better understanding of what your core value is, and therefore a better understanding of your true purpose in life—to manifest this value in the physical world. Try to think of a project or an activity that will allow this value to be expressed in all its glory, and write it down. This will be your seed for a better future.

CHAPTER 4

Ayurveda and Bhrigu Yoga

*He whose mind-body principles are in balance, whose
appetite is good, whose tissues are functioning
normally, whose waste products are in balance, and
whose body, mind and senses remain full of bliss, is
called a healthy person.*

–*Shushruta Samhita*, Sutrasthana *15:41*

Ayurveda—The Knowledge of Life

One day, at the Yoga Teacher Training Course in Ramat
Hasharon, Zipi brought her *Ayurveda* books, and the whole
lesson was dedicated to a discussion on *Ayurveda*. It was the
first time I had heard this term; it had a beautiful sound to it.

When Zipi explained the meaning of this term, my heart was
filled with joy, sensing I was close to finding new solutions
to many of my questions. She explained that *Ayurveda* is an
ancient Indian holistic and preventative approach to health,
literally meaning "knowledge of life" (*ayu* = life, *veda* =
knowledge). This body of knowledge dates back to 1500 BC

and includes all aspects of life from birth to death, including marriage, old age, family life, proper eating and sleeping habits, and much more. *Ayurveda* believes in nurturing healthy daily routines in order to create conditions for the whole body to be strong enough to heal itself and avoid diseases. It uses healthy foods and supplements in order to bring balance to the body, mind, emotions.

I found this idea to be revolutionary. This was a path that went hand in hand with yoga, and it could help us attain a more balanced life. Seeing the potential of this knowledge, I realized how it might impact our life by creating the conditions in which Arieldavid's body could heal itself. And creating these conditions required that I change as well. I began to see that helping Arieldavid to live a balanced life had inevitable implications for my own life. This understanding changed my outlook on life, bringing more enthusiasm, more interest, and curiosity.

Hearing Zipi talk about *Ayurveda*, I heard an inner voice say: "This is the path you need to follow; it holds all the answers for your quest to heal your son." And a year later, after completing the Integrated Yoga Teachers Training Course, I enrolled at Broshim Campus to study *Ayurveda*.

While studying *Ayurveda* I began to realize that my own life was being transformed as well, as a new path began to emerge in front of me. This path was parallel to the quest of healing Arieldavid, separate from it but intertwined at the same time. I realized that I was rewriting my own life story. What do I mean by rewriting?

Well, at that point, I was thirty-six years old and had been a practicing professional designer in the fields of furniture and exhibition design, as well as an academic lecturer. My whole identity was wrapped around my profession. I loved the design process that included everything from the idea of a meaningful esthetic object to its realization. My beliefs, wishes, and philosophy were all connected to my core belief that design could make people's lives better. Now, I was a student once again, studying anatomy and the different systems of the body according to *Ayurveda*. I was studying how to assist in the healing process of the body with natural herbs, a balanced daily routine (*Dinacharya*), body cleansing (*Pancha-Karma*), body strengthening with massage therapy (*Abhyanga*), and cooking. The latter included learning recipes and suitable compositions of foods, which bring balance to the three *Doshas* (human body types): *Vata*, *Pitta*, and *Kapha*. I quickly understood that theory is not enough to really learn this subject; I had to practice, be honest with myself, and observe my own way of life.

According to the book *Yoga Sutras of Patanjali*, my self-observation would be considered *"Svadhyaya,"* which is the fourth of five *Niyama* observances recommended by Patanjali. *Svadhyaya* is a Sanskrit word composed of "*Sva*," meaning "own, one's own self, the human soul," and "*Dhyana*," meaning "meditating on." The term *Svadhyaya*, therefore, also refers to "contemplation, reflection of oneself," or simply "to study one's own self."

In *Understanding Yoga Therapy*, Marlysa Sullivan describes *Svadhyaya* as a process in which the body becomes the representation of the teachings through which realization occurs. Here "*Sva*" means self, "*Dhy*" means absorption, and "*Ya*" means scriptures. *Svadhyaya* therefore signifies the manifestation of the scriptures through absorbing them into oneself to the point that they are apparent through one's actions. For me this was the actual goal, to be one with the teaching that resonated profoundly with my core value, "sanctify life."

My observations of my lifestyle and daily routine made me realize that I, too, needed to make changes in order to become more balanced. I discovered that to study something you believe in is one thing, but to actually live it is a much deeper level of understanding, and it is on that level that real change occurs. It is only there that you actually become the writer of your own life story as you learn how to think, act, and behave to such a degree that what you study, you become. I needed to live this Ayurvedic-yogic lifestyle if I really wanted my son to heal because I wanted to set an example for him. I believed that the change in me would make seem more natural to him the new lifestyle habits I was trying to incorporate.

In her book, Sullivan presents an insightful interpretation of Patanjali's commandments—the *Yamas* and *Niyamas*. She suggests applying *Svadhyaya*, or self-study, to daily life by developing a sense of nonjudgmental curiosity about oneself, one's beliefs, thoughts, emotions, behaviors, and interactions with others.

It was at that point that I was beginning to rewrite my life story parallel to helping my son to heal. I began to take care of my own health and daily routine, slowly transitioning from a lifestyle of a designer to a lifestyle of an *Ayurvedic* and yogic practitioner. This of course, is an ongoing, lifelong journey of adopting healthy habits and letting go of harmful ones, but after a few years, the changes were apparent, and I was able to witness many of my unhealthy habits transform into habits that supported my well-being.

Studying *Ayurveda* was a very big step in my son's healing process. It gave me an understanding of what he was going through. *Ayurveda*, from my own personal experience, is a very holistic, family-oriented way of living. It considers everything as part of a person's well-being: one's heritage, the way one lives, works, thinks, emotions, what a person eats, how the food is prepared, and when it is eaten. Even the way one prays is taken into consideration.

Broshim Campus has a unique characteristic in that it is designed to induce harmony. All the classes are on the ground floor and face the central garden. The environment is so peaceful that simply by being there and absorbing the air, my spirit was uplifted. I felt rejuvenated and empowered. Every week I looked forward to my daily studies there as this was an oasis for me.

Composing My Dinacharya

One of the fundamental *Ayurvedic* concepts that truly made an impact on my life, and as a result, on my son's life, was "*Dinacharya*," which in Sanskrit means "daily routine." Basically, *Dinacharya* is a compilation of recommendations of various daily actions and activities at specific times for sustaining a healthy lifestyle. In the book, *Textbook of Ayurveda, General Principles of Management and Treatment,* Dr. Vasant Lad explains the importance of *Dinacharya* as he writes: "Routine helps to establish balance in one's constitution. It also regularizes a person's biological clock, aids digestion, absorption, assimilation and generates self-esteem, discipline, peace, happiness and longevity."

In the beginning, when I first heard the concept of *Dinacharya*, I thought, "What is the big deal?" But after trying to bring some of the *Dinacharya* recommendations into my daily routine, I began to notice positive changes. My body loved the *Dinacharya*. It was as if it had found what it had always been looking for: a balanced lifestyle. The *Dinacharya* recommendations made perfect sense to my body, mind, and spirit.

I began to gradually change my daily routine to fit *Dinacharya's* recommendations. Some of these recommendations I wasn't able to incorporate into my life. Some changes took me years to assimilate. Others were a bit simpler, like going to sleep early. It was not easy to put away the work and the worries or even put my son to sleep earlier, but when it finally happened, it was an absolute blessing for me. Today I normally try to go to bed at around ten thirty, if not earlier, and I get up around five or five thirty. I find that this is a very good way to rejuvenate my body.

At that point, Arieldavid was seven years old. I was working a part-time job, but thanks to Adam's successful court appeals, we received another caregiver to help me look after him for a few hours a day, and I was finally able to go back to a full-time job, while keeping my role as a mother at the center of my life. As a busy working mom, it took some time to integrate meditation and yoga exercises into my daily life, but again, it was completely worthwhile when it finally happened. And pretty soon when I missed my morning yoga or meditation routine, I felt less resilient and experienced more stress throughout the day. On the days

I did practice, I had more energy and the ability to respond properly to the demands of that day.

As a mom to a child with a chronic condition, I know how important it is to create the best conditions for myself to be fit, strong, and happy to help my son heal and reach his fullest potential. By following *Dinacharya* and learning how to properly eat, sleep, and behave, I can actually harness the energy of nature and receive from it the support and balance I need.

This is the *Dinacharya* I composed for myself by tailoring the traditional *Dinacharya* suggestions to my personal needs. This simple daily routine helped me cultivate a balanced lifestyle for Arieldavid and me.

Morning

- Wake up early.
- Evacuate bowels and bladder.
- Once a week (sometimes more, in the fall and winter): self-*Abhyanga* (a gentle body massage with natural oils).
- Scrub tongue, brush teeth, and shower.
- Practice yoga postures (*asanas*).
- Chant mantras.
- Breathing exercises (*Pranayama*).

- Practice Storia Map meditation.
- Eat a light breakfast.
- Take Arieldavid to school.
- Go to work.

Afternoon

- Work.
- Eat lunch as the largest meal of the day.
- Pick up Arieldavid from school.
- Hike or playtime with Arieldavid.
- Work from home.

Evening

- Light stroll.
- Eat a light dinner before eight.
- Fun and relaxing activity with Arieldavid.
- Some form of meditation or relaxation like Yoga *Nidra* before bedtime.
- Quickly go over the day, saying thanks for the good things, resolving the things that went wrong.
- Visualize the next day according to our Storia Map.
- Go to bed early.

Finding a Jyotish

*Whatever happens is by His will and what seems
like free will really works by His power. The Almighty
returns to the good or evil fruits of their thoughts and
deeds in earlier bodies. It is best to accept His will,
but one will not tremble under sorrows if one looks to
Him for the strength to endure them.*

**–Shri Sudhir Rnajan Bhadury, also known
as Sudhi Babu, from "A Search in Secret India"
by Paul Brunton**

Arieldavid was nearly seven years old when I approached
the end of my second year of *Ayurveda* studies at Broshim
Campus in Tel Aviv. We were practicing many *Ayurveda*
techniques and recommendations at home and were
able to balance and sustain his health. However, he was
still ventilated all the time, unable to disconnect from the
machine for more than a few minutes without the oxygen
levels in his blood dropping to harmful levels, putting his
life at risk.

My son's loving eyes and huge smile spoke to my heart.
I felt restless. I could not find peace while he was in this
state. "There will be a way," I continued to say to him,
"In my mind, you're already healed, living a full and happy
life."

I continued to pray for him, yet this was not becoming a reality. "What else can I do?" I asked myself and, filled with hope, turned to *Ayurveda*. I found that according to the *Ayurveda* scriptures, the cause of any disease is rooted in the spirit and manifests itself on the physical level in the body as a symptom. So in order to heal the root of the problem, the spiritual struggle has to be resolved.

Intuitively I felt that my son was undergoing some kind of spiritual issue that I couldn't fathom. I felt that he was experiencing an energetic block that would not let his body heal. But I didn't really know what this meant or even how to approach this. What do you do when you have tried everything but still cannot overcome the problem?

The next day, during *Ayurveda* class, I asked one of my teachers this question.

"It seems like your solution can only be found by a *Jyotish*," she answered.

"What is a *Jyotish*? And where do I find one?" I asked.

"A *Jyotish* is someone who can open the energy flow when the energy is blocked somewhere in the body," she replied, "You can find a *Jyotish* in India, but it is very hard to find a true *Jyotish*."

I was very happy to hear this hopeful news, and regardless of being a bit upset to hear that this might be a very difficult task, I was suddenly overwhelmed by thoughts about how I could get to India and where I would look if I managed to get there.

The next morning, an internal knowing directed me to do the only thing I could do: SURRENDER. I knew I had reached a point where I could do nothing more than to offer my prayer to God and let him provide a solution. I did not go to class that morning, and instead of taking the bus to Tel-Aviv, I took the bus in the other direction to Jerusalem. The only person who knew where I was going was my classmate and good friend, Tomer.

The entire way to Jerusalem, I formulated my prayer to find a *Jyotish* and hoped with all my heart that God would hear me. The bus station was packed as I reached Jerusalem. People from all over the world were going about their business. I was struck by the immense diversity I saw whenever I turned to look on my way to the old city in Jerusalem. It made me think of the greatness of God, who has created so many unique flowers. Surely this great God could help me find a *Jyotish* to help save one of those beautiful flowers. I could not do this on my own any longer, I thought. I needed guidance to reach the next step of my son's well-being and livelihood.

I reached the holy house of prayer and entered. Sitting to my right and left were two other women who were praying wholeheartedly. I sat down and began to pray. I don't know how much time passed as I was completely absorbed by my prayer and lost contact with my surroundings, holding a single intention in my mind.

"Please, God, send me a *Jyotish* to heal my son," I repeated again and again. After some time, I regained awareness of my surroundings, and I felt calm. Not sad or anxious. Simply calm. A certainty that everything would work out had fallen upon me. It felt like the wings of an angel had lifted my burden off of my heart and healed me like a lost child, giving me peaceful comfort in knowing that everything, somehow, would be all right.

Upon leaving the house of prayer, I reached for my phone to check for any messages and to my astonishment, I had received a message from Tomer, saying, "You are not going to believe this. Return as soon as you can to Campus Broshim. They have just announced in class that an unexpected guest lecturer is coming tonight. He is an *Ayurvedic* doctor accompanied by his brother, a *Vedic Jyotish*; they arrived from Varanasi, India."

I was amazed, ecstatic, and grateful. I rushed back to the bus stop to return to Tel-Aviv.

When the Student is Ready,
the Teacher Appears

On my way back to Tel-Aviv from Jerusalem, I was contemplating the remarkable circumstances that had brought me to meet this *Jyotish*. The old saying, "When the student is ready, the teacher appears" was ringing in my mind. "But what do I expect him to do?" I asked myself. "What can he teach me?" And what about the *Ayurvedic* doctor that was giving the lecture? What could I learn from him?

The one word that kept coming to me was SURRENDER. *What am I to surrender to?* I tried to debate with my inner voice. But there was no answer, only the same word: SURRENDER. But I could not surrender to what I did not know or understand.

I reached Tel-Aviv just in time. As I entered the class in Campus Broshim, I saw people already sitting and waiting. The room was packed, and I felt lucky I got a good spot close to the front row.

After a few minutes, the lecturer arrived, accompanied by his family and close students.

A faculty member of the Ayurveda department of Campus Broshim introduced the speaker as Dr. Jayant Kumar

Bhadury, an *Ayurvedic* doctor from Varanasi, India, a master yogi in *Bhrigu* yoga, and a *Brahman* (high priest).

Dr. Bhadury began his talk by first introducing his wife, Vatsala Bhadury, his twin brother, Acharya Hemant Kumar Bhadury, a *Vedic Jyotish*, and his wife, Mithlesh Kishori Bhadury. He explained that the four of them worked very closely together, using *mantras*, *yantras*, and energy to help people purify and balance the body and mind. He added that everything they knew was passed to them from his father and mother, Shri Shri Dr. Brahma Gopal Bhadury and Shri Mati Dr. Rita Bhadury. Their father, the great guru Shri Dr. Brahma Gopal Bhadury Mahasaya, was known as a sage and a yogi that mastered the secrets of *Jyotish*, *Tantra*, *Ayurveda*, yoga, and philosophy. He was considered a great *Tantric Kaulachari* (a rare stream of knowledge that makes use of the beneficial powers of *Tantra* and hidden forces that cure diseases and bring prosperity and happiness).

Dr. Brahma Gopal Bhadury received this ancient knowledge from his father and mother, Shri Shri Sudhi Ranjan Bhadury and Kalyani Devi. Shri Sudhir Ranjan Bhadury (also known as Sudhi Babu) was a great yogi born in 1880 to the royal Bengali Brahmin family (in Nabadvip), Nadia district in West Bengal. After graduating school, he renounced his royal wealth for the pursuit of spiritual- and self-realization while being a family man in Varanasi.

I thought it was remarkable to be part of such a spiritual yet practical lineage. What a wonderful thing to be able to teach your children how to balance the body and mind and live harmoniously with the world while helping others.

Dr. Bhadury began to speak about cancer and how to treat it from the point of view of *Ayurveda*. He also introduced some *Bhrigu* yoga exercises to improve health and create balance.

During the lecture, I felt as if time had stopped moving, but my mind was racing with thoughts. What exactly should I ask Dr. Bhadury and his brother the *Jyotish*? Could they be the answer to my prayers? How could they help when Arieldavid and I were here in Israel, and they lived in India? I received no answer to these questions or to the ones that followed.

After a few minutes of contemplating what I should do, I realized that I had no choice except to surrender to whatever was about to come. To surrender to a higher power, knowing that everything would be as it should, knowing that everything I had done for the past eight years had led me to this moment where I needed to take another leap of faith toward the unknown. "It's okay. Don't worry," I said to myself. "Your prayer has been answered; now simply relax and listen." My mind finally settled down.

The lecture went on for about an hour. When it ended, I approached Dr. Bhadury to ask him for his guidance on my quest to heal my son. Dr. Bhadury listened to me attentively, and after I finished explaining the background of our situation, he suggested that I meet with him and his brother for a private session the following day at the home he and his family were staying in, where for the following days, he and his brother were meeting people for private consultations, giving readings of astrology maps for them, and giving advice and guidance on how to improve their lives through the application of *Bhrigu* yoga and *Ayurveda*.

Written in the Stars

The next morning, I reached the address I had been given. Dr. Bhadury's wife, Vatsala Ji, greeted me, and we spoke about Arieldavid for a few minutes until Dr. Bhadury was free to meet me.

When I met Dr. Bhadury and he began to speak, I was deeply moved by his peaceful tone of voice. I had never heard someone speak in such a calm tone before. There was detachment in his words, but at the same time, there was an attentive caring. He seemed to say things as they were, with clarity and simplicity. It was clear that he genuinely wanted to help my son and me to have a better life.

Dr. Bhadury shared with me some of the possibilities that his brother, Acharya Hemant K. Bhadury, saw in the reading of my astrological map. He explained that these were only possibilities and not a definite reality. He recommended things I should avoid and good habits I should adopt. He shared with me some mantras to balance the mind and body. I also met with his brother, the *Jyotish*, who shared with me the difficulties my son had gone through in previous years, which he could see in his astrological map, which I confirmed. He spoke about one of Arieldavid's possible futures as well, which gave me hope. He emphasized that in order to actualize this possibility, I would need to make a lot of effort to help my son. I said that it was my wish to assist with Arieldavid's growth, health, and development, and I would do whatever I could to help him.

Talking to Dr. Bhadury and Acharya Bhadury helped me to ease my worried heart. I felt reassured that I was headed in the right direction.

"Come again tomorrow, and we will do something for your son," Dr. Bhadury added at the end of our meeting.

I returned the next morning, excited with anticipation. When I entered the house, again, I was astonished by how much peace there was in the presence of Dr. Bhadury, Vatsala Ji, Dr. Bhadury's brother, and his wife. It was inspiring to see how calm they all were, considering the many things that they were doing: meeting people, giving lectures, holding consultations, etc.

How are they so peaceful? I, too, would like to be so peaceful, especially in the midst of a busy day, I thought to myself. *Is it possible for a mother like me to live a full life, help her son reach his fullest potential, and remain peaceful all at the same time?* I asked myself as I was invited to sit down in the living room and wait for Dr. Bhadury to meet with me.

As I waited for Dr. Bhadury, his wife Vatsala Ji kept me company. We spoke about Arieldavid, and I showed her some photos of him. She then smiled and told me a wonderful folktale. It was a story about a young boy who had special needs. His mother was tending to him, and one day, she heard a knock on her door. She opened the door, and a *Sadu* (a holy man who devotes himself to God while giving up all his worldly positions) was standing there with his hand held out toward her as if asking for food or money.

Though she was a poor woman, the boy's mother was a strong believer in God and in her duties as a devotee, and thus she said, "I don't have food to give you or money as we are very poor, but, if you wish, I can draw water from our well for you."

The *Sadu* nodded his head in agreement, and they both set out to the backyard, where the well was located. She began to pull up the rope, and the bucket appeared with water in it. She handed the bucket to the *Sadu*, who drank the water with much vigor as he was very thirsty. After he finished, he thanked her and added, "I saw you have a young boy at home with special needs. See how this rope has changed the form of the stone against which it repeatedly grinds, creating a channel in it? The same will be true for your son. If you teach him repeatedly, eventually he will learn and change."

Hearing this folktale was very encouraging to me. Even though I already knew this concept, it was still reassuring to hear it from another point of view and culture. For me, the moral of this story is **to do**. It's not enough to believe in something. One must actually do things, over and over again, in order to turn faith into a reality, even if it seems impossible.

Dr. Bhadury came in and asked me to follow him into a smaller room, where his brother was sitting as well. I spoke with both of them about my deep wish for my son to heal and live a full life, and they listened attentively. I was very grateful that we had been able to sustain Arieldavid's life up to this point, but I wished for him much more out of life, to be free from the ventilation machine, and to be able to run and play outside like other children his age.

When I finished talking, they spoke with each other in Hindi, and after a few minutes, they seemed to have reached an understanding. "We can do a *Puja* for your son," Acharya Bhadury said.

"What is a *Puja*? What does it do? And when can we start?" I asked.

They explained that a *Puja* is a special prayer directed toward the health, balance, happiness and overall well-being of the individual the *Puja* is done for. It is performed by a trained priest who chants a special mantra around three thousand times a day, for about eight hours a day, for forty-two consecutive days, which total up to one hundred and thirty-seven thousand, five hundred mantras. These mantras are supposed to energetically purify the spiritual channel of the person receiving the *Puja* in order to help that person's natural life force to rejuvenate itself so that energy may flow harmoniously in the body, helping to restore health and balance to the individual.

This was exactly what I was looking for—some kind of a procedure that would clean the spiritual blockages in Arieldavid's life and boost his overall development. "Yes, let's do it!" I said. "When can we begin the *Puja*?"

"Come tomorrow," they replied.

Arieldavid's Puja

The next morning, I returned to start Arieldavid's *Puja*. I was shown into a small room, where Dr. Bhadury was sitting on the floor with his legs crossed. Acharya Bhadury sat by his side. I was asked to join them and sat on the floor across from them. Vatsala Ji put a few grains of rice and a few drops of water in my right palm and a coin in the left palm. They spoke with someone on the phone in Hindi. They explained that this was the priest who would perform the daily mantras from the temple located at their home in Varanasi.

After a few minutes I was asked by them to say my son's name out loud, which I did. After a few seconds, I heard the man on the other end of the line begin to chant a mantra. I was told it was in Sanskrit. I heard the man chanting my son's name. I felt as if my mind was transported into another dimension. I felt relaxed and calm. I felt that things were already changing for the better. I felt my son was changing as well. It was not something I could explain in words, but internally, it felt real to me.

Two years after the *Puja* was performed for Arieldavid, my son's condition substantially improved. Finally, after being ventilated almost all hours of the day and night, we were gradually able to disconnect him from the ventilation machine to the point where he was breathing independently for most of his waking hours.

There was no medical explanation for this improvement, and for me, it was a clear result of the energy cleansing done on Arieldavid's channels. For me it was a miracle that I attributed to God, to the Bhadury family, and to the *Puja* that eventually allowed this miracle to take place. Thanks to the *Puja*, the events unfolded in the direction of healing and improvement in the life quality of Arieldavid, and at the age of ten, he was finally breathing independently in all his waking hours during the day and enjoying his life as a kid.

I am forever grateful for what Dr. Bhadury and his family have done for my son and me. It marked the beginning of a long-term relationship that continues to this very day. A relationship that began as a consultation and developed into me becoming a student of *Bhrigu* yoga and choosing Dr. Bhadury as my guru, spiritual guide, and yoga teacher for the path of self-realization and living a pure life while as a family woman.

Today it is my personal aim to let other people know about this amazing family and the deep knowledge they hold in aiding people and improving the quality of life, health, and happiness through the daily practice of *Bhrigu* yoga, chanting mantras, yantras, and keeping a daily routine that promotes purity and good family life.

If you, too, want to learn more about the Bhadury family, the yogi lineage they come from, and the unique knowledge they offer, you can read all about them on their website, www.bhrigu.yoga.

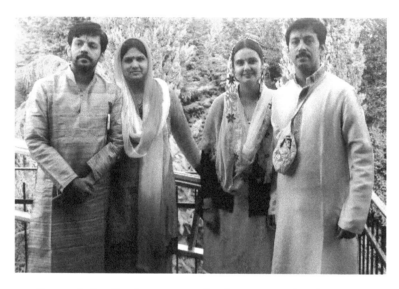

From right: Dr. Jayant K. Bhadury, Vatsala Bhadury,
Mithlesh Kishori Bhadury, and
Acharya Hemant K. Bhadury, 2019

The Farmer's Meditation

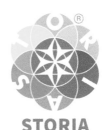

STORIA

Overview: **The proverb "As you sow, so shall you reap" means that our future is shaped by our present thoughts, intentions, and actions. The Farmer's Meditation is a powerful meditation that leverages this idea in order to manifest** the future we desire. Our intention holds the very seed of whatever future event or experience we would like to create. Thus, we need to choose our seeds very carefully so that they may yield the trees that bear the fruit we wish to relish in the future. So please, try to be aware of your thoughts, as the mind creates what it imagines, even if we're not aware of it. Knowing that, it is reckless to let negativity seep into our mind—into the seat of creation. Instead, we should choose our thoughts very carefully, consciously constructing our vision of a meaningful and healthy life for ourselves, our families, and our communities.

It is here, in this meditation, that you may choose to take an active role in fulfilling your dreams and making the changes you have always wanted. In this setting, you orient yourself toward writing the new chapter of your life, which will, eventually, manifest as an entirely new and exciting life story. It all begins with choosing the good seeds and planting them in the fertile soil of your mind. For this purpose, you may use as your seeds the core values you have discerned in the "My Life's Exhibition" exercise in the previous chapter.

Preparation

Set the place for your meditation. Take time to prepare it, as this is a sacred place.

The place should be clean and quiet. You may also want to light a small candle and incense (sandalwood is always recommended). Turn off your phone and other electronic devices for the next fifteen minutes as you invest this time in yourself. Sit comfortably in an upright position on a yoga mat, a pillow, or a chair. Close your eyes softly, inhale deeply through your nose, and slowly exhale through your mouth. Relax yourself more and more with every breath you take, feeling the weight of your own body as your awareness expands in all directions, beyond your body's outline.

Steps

1. Your Marvelous Land

   Imagine you are standing in front of a marvelous piece of land filled with flower beds of beautiful, dark, fertile earth. This fertile land is your subconscious, filled with all possibilities, ready to manifest any future you desire.

2. **Pulling out the Weeds**

   As you begin to walk on this magical land, looking around in wonder, you notice something. You see that there are weeds growing in the earth, draining it of precious potential energy. These weeds are your limiting beliefs, your negative thoughts and convictions, which prevent you from growing. Try to identify a few of them. See them clearly in front of you. Get closer. Pull them carefully out of the ground and put them in a sack. Make sure you pluck the weeds from the root up so that they won't bother you any longer. Repeat this process until the land looks clean enough and ready for seeding.

3. **Choosing the Seeds**

   Take a deep breath and relax. Take a few moments to think about the seeds you will need in order to have the fruits you desire. It could be that you want a better relationship with your partner, which may require the seed of understanding, or maybe you need the seed of forgiveness to find peace in your heart, or perhaps it is the seed of gratitude that will enable you to appreciate what your partner is already giving you. Whatever you truly want to manifest in your life, consider what needs to happen and what actions you are required to take.

When you have an idea of what you would like to plant in the fertile soil of your unconscious mind, simply turn to your right. There you will find a bag with a label reading "Good Seeds." These seeds contain within them the genetic code for the future you wish to experience, which includes all the right opportunities, resources, useful habits, people, attitudes, and anything else you might need on your journey.

Note: If you completed the "My Life's Exhibition" exercise from the previous chapter, you might have already realized your life's values for the future you want to manifest. If this is the case, you may choose these values as the "Good Seeds" in this part of the meditation. If you have not done this exercise, or if you have, but feel other seeds will be more helpful in this moment in your life, it is perfectly fine to go ahead and choose the seeds you need.

4. Planting the Good Seeds

    Start walking down the flower beds, and plant your good seeds along the path. Every time you do this, bless the seeds as you plant them in the soil. See in your mind's eye how the seeds you are so thoughtfully planting will grow into magnificent trees with succulent fruits. See how these fruits will be distributed to future generations in twenty-five years, fifty years, a hundred years, and even in two hundred years. Know without a doubt that your efforts, as pioneering as they might be, will produce the change you want to see in the world, even if this will be in a time that you, physically, will not get to witness. Just the internal instinct, the knowing in itself, will bring much satisfaction to your heart. Cherish this moment before walking back to the entrance of the field.

5. The Bonfire and the Rain

Now, return to the entrance of the field and make a big bonfire near the entrance, putting the weeds in the fire to energetically release your soul and land from them so that you may embark on a new journey and make a fresh start. See how, as the smoke goes up into the sky, it summons the rain, which pours over the field, blessing it with purity and life. Take a deep breath and see the field you've planted in a new light, like a mother looking at her newborn, blessing this newcomer for the very first time with a happy, healthy, full life.

Conclusion

Take a deep breath and slowly open your eyes. Congratulate yourself for creating this beautiful experience using your own willpower and imagination. By rehearsing this, you will create the steps needed to reach the future you long for.

CHAPTER 5

The Storia Map

If you treat an individual as he is, he will remain how he is. But if you treat him as if he were what he ought to be and could be, he will become what he ought to be and could be.

— Johann Wolfgang Von Goethe

Arieldavid's Future Portrait

In a small book called *Silence as Yoga,* Swami Paramananda describes the process of looking within to find the connection between the creator and oneself. Paramananda writes:

> In India, they adopt the simple practice that before they eat, drink, study, go to sleep or undertake any business, they sit in silence for a moment and try to unite themselves with the center of their being. When we are distracted by outer conditions or concerns, we lose our sense of proportion and we cannot do what we have to do. As long as our physical eyes lead us to see the many, we cannot

see the one; so the devotee closes his outer eyes
that he may open his inner eye and with it, perceive
the deeper realities within. He closes his outer ears
that he may hear the voice of infinity in his heart.

These words take me to my own inner vision, a vision that
entered my mind and heart fifteen years ago when my son
was born. A vision that has not left me since and has only
grown and developed into a detailed visual story of how
my son healed and now lives a full and happy life. This clear
inner vision gave me one direction to follow, no matter
what was going on at the time. It was like a beam of light
extending into the dark night and showing me the way
home.

There was nothing else in my mind except this one vision
of Arieldavid, all grown up, in his teens, healed, happy,
living a full life, and from then on, living happily and fully
throughout his life. This clear vision cut through all doubt
caused by the obstacles we were facing in the first years of
his life.

As I held the image steady in my mind, I was empowered and
woke up every morning with a clear purpose to continue
moving forward in my attempt to stabilize, balance, and
strengthen my son's health and develop his cognitive,
emotional, and physical well-being. This vision gave me the
perseverance and the courage I needed when facing crises
and emergencies. It gave me the resilience and patience

throughout the many years it took to see a substantial positive change in Arieldavid's quality of life. This vision provided me with hope as I focused not on what was missing in my son's life, but more importantly and more effectively, on what his life might become. But how could I present this vision to my son? Was there a way for me to bring my vision of him to life, so he could witness it as well?

A portrait! I thought enthusiastically. *That would be the perfect solution.*

For over nine years, I had known about Massimo's paintings, as I had first seen his work in Le Case near Assisi, where I participated in my first retreat. His paintings covered the wall of the hallway that led to the meditation hall, as if to mentally prepare the retreat participants before entering. I personally believed Massimo had a rare ability to convey an idea in such a way that anyone who looked at his work could feel the feeling he tried to evoke. This is sometimes termed "objective art"; the ability to create the desired shift in the viewer's mindset and emotions, preferably toward some useful emotions, as well as a more balanced mind.

He would be perfect for the job, I thought. Excited, I searched for a way to contact him. Once I found his email, I sent him a message, and we scheduled an online Skype meeting to discuss the commission for the painting.

"Hi!" I uttered to Massimo, feeling self-conscious and uncomfortable about the request I was about to make, out of fear it might sound crazy. "Can you paint my son's portrait?"

Massimo replied with a smile, "Yes, of course." He seemed like a gentle man in his mid-fifties. Still, as I was about to explain exactly what I wanted, I felt my initial bit of confidence was wearing off. *How can he possibly understand me? How can he see what is in my heart and bring it to life on a canvas? He will think I am crazy!* I thought. "Oh, relax," I said to my insecurity. "You can do this. Just ask him. You have waited for so long to be able to communicate this image to your son, and this painter is capable of doing that. He is a master painter."

My thoughts were interrupted by Massimo's next question: "Can you send me a picture of your son?"

"Yes and no," I said. "You see, I need you to paint my son in the future, the way he will be or could be, or to be more accurate, the way I see him in the future."

Massimo looked confused. "I do not understand," he said.

I paused, trying to figure out how to explain this. Even though I had thought of this before, when I actually needed to speak, I got cold feet. "Have courage, Yamina. Have courage," I said to myself as I closed my eyes for a moment.

"My son is going to be eleven years old soon, and he has only recently begun to breathe on his own during most of his waking hours," I said without looking directly into the computer screen. "You see, he was born with a rare, life-threatening condition of not having an automatic breathing command. However, since he was born, I have seen him in my mind's eye healthy, happy, independent, traveling the world, bringing hope to people with similar circumstances, loved by all, and living a full life."

Tears were rolling down my cheeks, which I hoped Massimo did not see as I felt self-conscious and exposed. Here I was, talking with a complete stranger about my deepest wishes that I shared with only a few very close people. I was afraid he would dismiss my concept or think I was out of my mind.

"And," I continued, "I want to find a way to share with him my vision of him being healthy, happy, and living a full life. I want to convey to him that he is not his illness, that he is not the body, that he is who he sees himself as being, and not what anyone else says."

I stopped to catch my breath. "You see, I have been carrying this hope internally for so long— more than ten years—and we have gone through so much pain, trauma, and so much suffering. I just want him to know that no matter what happens, I always believed in him and believed that God will find the way to help us."

I paused again and, after taking a deep breath, I said, "I'm not crazy. My son is the love of my life, and I made him a promise the day he was born. I promised him that he would have an amazing life no matter what and that, God willing, he would be healed. Will you help me with a painting that represents my vision?" I asked Massimo and raised my head to meet his eyes on the other side of the screen.

Now it was Massimo who was crying, and this time he was the one talking with downcast eyes. "You are an incredible mother," he said softly. "Yes, I will help you. How do you see him in the future? I have never done such a portrait before, so I need to understand what you see."

Overwhelmed by his positive response, I quickly replied, "I don't know yet exactly. I need to think more about the scenery. I only know that my son loves to travel, so it would be wonderful for the setting to be somewhere in nature. Perhaps it can even be in the hillsides of Umbria, overlooking Assisi, where my internal vision and personal direction was strengthened by the example of Saint Francis's wall painting of his stigmata."

"Very well," Massimo replied, "Send me a photo of your son today, and I will see how I can paint him as he could be ten years from now, at the age of twenty-one."

Several weeks went by as Massimo sent me examples of his interpretation of my vision. My request was detailed, but many things were left to Massimo's imagination. I began to see Massimo as a kind of a magician, because his depiction of how I saw my son was very precise. It seemed as if he connected with my son's energy and my own in order to bring this vision to life on the canvas. It was an amazing, magical process for me to witness. Toward the completion of Arieldavid's future portrait, I noticed that Massimo gave Arieldavid a cane to hold, so I asked him about it.

"It's because he is a teacher," he answered, "and one day may lead many others. A cane is a symbol; it is representing someone who is leading others."

I was very moved by his words. *Yes,* I thought to myself, *He is a teacher, my teacher. His mere presence is the teaching. He teaches by example that even in the harshest conditions, it is possible to live a life of kindness, happiness, courage, perseverance, gratitude, and find joy in the little things. And maybe one day he will be able to speak about it as well and share his knowledge with others.*

I was very grateful and uplifted; I could not have asked for a better artist and human than Massimo to paint Arieldavid's self-portrait.

A few months had gone by when the completed portrait arrived at our home. Filled with excitement, I watched my son attentively as he opened the parcel. We rolled out the canvas, and there was the portrait of my son in the future, looking straight into his own face.

The future is already here, I thought to myself, tears of joy rolling down my cheeks. Arieldavid seemed very happy. He was smiling with gratitude, and I knew that a part of him understood that this was him as he could be one day.

From that day on, there has not been one day that I have not looked at Arieldavid's portrait and asked myself what more I can do to make this intention a reality. It has become a focal part of our daily practice, a reminder of where we are headed. Each day, at the end of our daily yoga practice, Arieldavid points to the painting, and I verbalize to him his Storia Map that this image represents. I say out loud what I see as he smiles and shakes his hands in excitement. "With God's help, Arieldavid is strong, healthy, happy, and is breathing independently, traveling the world with our family, teaching yoga, and bringing peace, hope, and joy to people through his incredible story."

Arieldavid loves this part of our practice, and I do too. This is more than a story; this is an affirmation I put out into the universe. This affirmation has a long-term impact on the ideas and actions I take. The portrait has become a way for me to remind my son of how his life quality might greatly improve, and his cooperation is vital for its success.

I will forever be grateful to Massimo for agreeing to paint my son's portrait in the future, as it has been and still is a powerful tool for me to help Arieldavid see himself in a different and positive light. To see himself as a healed and fulfilled young man, as I do in my mind's eye. Then I can talk to him about a specific action we can do together to help him reach this state and ask him if he is willing to take the next step.

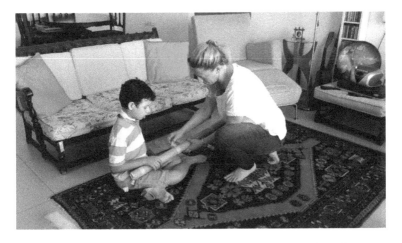

Arieldavid and Yamina opening the parcel with
Arieldavid's portrait, 2015

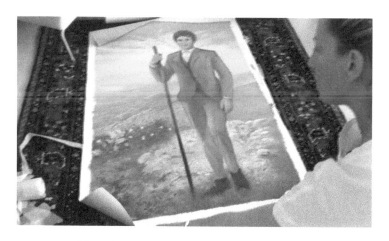

Arieldavid and Yamina looking at Arieldavid's portrait, 2015

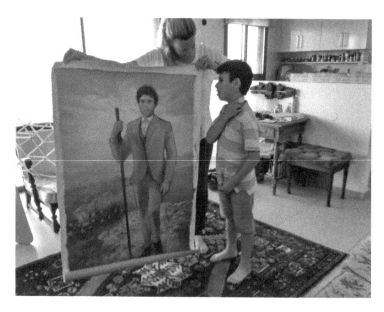

Arieldavid and Yamina looking at Arieldavid's portrait, 2015

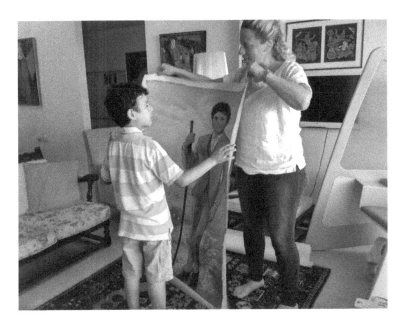

Arieldavid and Yamina looking at Arieldavid's
portrait, 2015

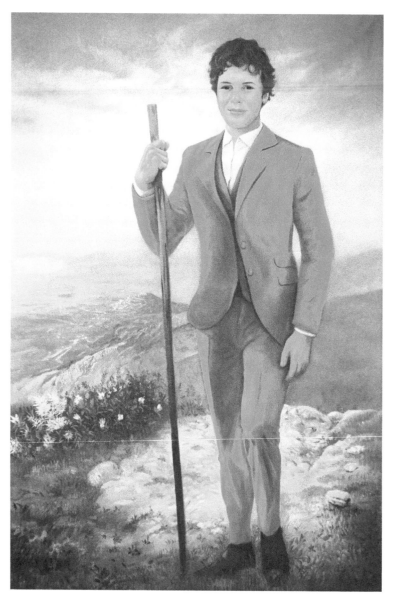

Arieldavid's portrait in the future, 2015

Creating the Storia Map

The Creative Power within us makes us into the image of that to which we give our attention... In order to do this, man must pass from the competitive to the creative mind; he must form a clear mental picture of the things he wants, and hold this picture in his thoughts with the fixed PURPOSE to get what he wants, and the unwavering FAITH that he does get what he wants, closing his mind to all that may tend to shake his purpose, dim his vision, or quench his faith. That he may receive what he wants when it comes, man must act NOW upon the people and things in his present environment.

–The Science of Getting Rich *by Wallace D. Wattles*

What would you do if you knew where you wanted to go but did not know how to get there?

Where would you look? And how would you start your quest? You would most likely need a map that would take you from your location to the designated point. This was the reason I created Storia Map, to help Arieldavid and me navigate through the challenges we faced and reach our goal.

Many people today are aware of the concept that you attract what you think about, and so you can intentionally create the reality you desire. However, a lot of the time, for some reason, we still create the opposite of what we want. This is due to the fact that, unknowingly, we still host a lot of unwanted negative thoughts and emotions in our mind. Most of the time we are not really in control; our thoughts are contradictory, random, and scattered, and each one pulls us in a different direction, preventing us from moving decisively in the direction we want. The more that your body, mind, and speech are aligned, and the more that your thoughts, emotions, words, and actions communicate and cooperate in trying to achieve the same objective, the faster you will be able to attract what you really want.

This is where Storia comes in. The Storia Map helps to align and unify all of your scattered parts by shedding light, specifying, and organizing the different aspects of your life that together make up the whole. In this way, the map bridges the vision you have with the reality you are currently experiencing, creating a clear path of how to manifest your dream.

To this day, I have kept very close to my heart my internal image of Arieldavid healed, and I refer back to it several times a day, drawing energy, strength, and hope from it. It's not difficult; in fact, I believe it's a simple process that anyone can do. It relieves the stress I am feeling and relaxes me. This image of my son healed and happy makes me very glad indeed. All I have to do is merely ask for the image of a better life for him, and the rest will naturally appear by itself. This image is the core of the Storia Map.

The name I chose for this method is "Storia," which has a double meaning in Italian: the first meaning is "history," and the second is "story." I like the double meaning because, for me, it symbolizes that no matter what your history is, the future is yet to be told, and only you, with God's grace, can create the life story you envision.

The next step was charting the Storia Map sections for Arieldavid based on what he needed and wanted. By observing him, I could understand him and his needs and adjust his map accordingly. The things that made him happy gave me the deepest insight and allowed me to tap into what he really wanted. I could then create a plan and integrate it into a visual map to help me stay on the right path. This might sound simplified, but in fact it is a deep process of getting to understand yourself and/or another person's interests, likes, dislikes, and the ability to learn what is required to manifest your vision.

Charting the Storia Map in Four Steps

Step 1: A Wishful Image

Every Storia Map begins with an image.

The image of the desired future is the core of the Storia Map, and for a very good reason—our mind and emotions respond much better to images than to words or other mediums. There is a significant amount of research that proves that visualization can help in improving emotional states, supporting healing processes and enhancing athletic performance.

I didn't know this at the time; for me it happened intuitively. The image, for me, was the engine behind all my actions. I had in my mind's eye, from the very beginning of his life, the image of my son healed completely, happy, beautiful, and radiating livelihood. I could see him, internally, sitting on a bench, surrounded by nature, smiling and laughing full-heartedly. In time, this image developed to include other events and activities. The more I imagined, the more I saw them manifest in reality. And the more I saw the changes in reality, the easier it was to imagine and develop more of our Storia Map.

It is like telling a story with pictures about how you would like your life to be in the future, only you're telling this story as if it has already happened or is happening in the present moment, regardless of the actual circumstances. It's important to hold the image patiently, decisively, for as long as it takes, until you manifest the reality that is so significant to you.

This visualization process corresponds with the Jewish saying: "Every action begins with thought," which means that before you can deliberately act, you must have an idea of what the action is going to be. This also means that whatever you experience has its roots in thought, for better and for worse. This is a rule to live by because it puts your destiny in your own hands as you become a cocreator of your reality and not merely a spectator. So when you visualize, it is like you're saying to the universe, "Hey, down here. I am here, and this...Yes, this is what I want."

So let's try it together. Simply close your eyes for a moment and try to relax while holding the intention for a better life. Your heart's wishes will effortlessly begin to rise up to your consciousness, and an image will begin to appear in your mind's eye. Let the image surface up in a natural way, without any force, but rather from a place of deep relaxation. When the images start to surface, observe them like a movie. Notice if there are movements, colors, and things you may or may not recognize. The more you let your imagination run freely, the more the images will resonate with your inner self, and you will be energized.

In the beginning, it might seem unreasonable that this image will manifest itself. Maybe it will look like "a happy ending movie" that has no bearing on your current situation. My advice? Enjoy the ride. Let this movie take you up and lift your spirit. There is a famous quote by Albert Einstein: "Imagination is more important than knowledge." He is right! When constructing the Storia Map, keep out indecisiveness, doubt, judgment, and regret. Let yourself imagine without any constraints while holding the intention to see a better future for yourself, your family, and your community.

My own experience with this thought process is that behind a meaningful thought, there is a deep wish that resides in the heart. So, when I visualize, I feel the energy of my heart bring up the image in my mind's eye. Once you have this initial core image, you can develop it even further to make it more precise and vivid.

Think about your desired reality and try to see the different aspects that it entails. Try to construct your wishful image by answering the following questions, giving you an in-depth perspective into your wishful image as a whole:

- **Body** – What does your body look like? How does it feel? How does it reflect who you want to become?

- **Mind** – What are your thoughts like? Their quality? The interests? Where is your attention directed?

- **Emotions** – Which emotions do you most frequently host within you? Do they give you strength and motivation?

- **Giving (Out)** – What are you creating in your life? Are you able to share these fruits with others?

- **Behavior** – How does the person you wish to become behave in different situations? How does he/she react to unpleasant stimulations?

- **Receiving (In)** – What gifts might you receive? How will they all allow you to grow? Personally? Spiritually? Economically?

Try to answer these questions with as much detail as possible and see these details as part of your image. The more effort and thought you put in, the clearer and more powerful your image will become. When you feel satisfied with the result, you can move on to the next step of creating your Storia Map.

Note: Don't worry if the image is not fully vivid yet; you can always return to this section to develop and expand this vision.

Step 2: The Practical Method

Now that we clearly see where we are going, we need to find the best route to get there. This route is the method, the means by which we will get to our destination. The method doesn't have to be complex; in fact it should be very simple and straightforward. It should be a simple procedure or an action that you can repeat almost daily, until it becomes a habit. Most importantly it should stem from your image, meaning that every time you follow this method, it should bring you a little bit closer to your desired reality.

Keep in mind that the changes will not always be apparent within short time frames, so it's important to stay positive and patient. By trusting yourself and this process, you will receive the strength and resilience you need. It took ten years until I saw my son breathing on his own during the daytime. If I had given up on believing that one day he would heal, I would never have been able to look for the methods that helped him to reach this reality.

Therefore, the method that you choose, for whatever length of time you feel you may try it, needs to have your complete faith and dedication. In our case, the main method was and still is yoga. But it took me several years of trying different methods, parallel to yoga, until I found it to be my core method, my fire and fuel to continue to aim to reach my dreams for my son's well-being and, with time, to include myself in them as well.

In order to find the right method for you, I highly recommend that you follow these steps:

- **Research** – Be open-minded and look for an answer anywhere you can think of. Try to find methods that are scientifically proven to work or at least that have worked for others. Seek advice from people that already went through what you're going through or who have already achieved a similar goal.

- **Experiment** – Try out some of these methods and see what works for you. Stay in touch with your intuition and notice which methods appeal to you more than others. Give each method a fair amount of time and dedication before you move on to the next one. And don't try them all at once.

- **Gather Feedback and Statistics** – Be open-minded, but don't follow blindly. Be aware of any changes this method is producing, and use this feedback to tweak this method for your needs or to drop it altogether if you see that it doesn't work for you after a sufficient period of time.

You could say that this step is basically a recap from Chapter 3. You may remember that in Chapter 3, I shared with you one of the first variations of the Storia Map. This map was basically a list of methods divided into categories. I knew what I wanted, and I saw it clearly in my mind's eye—I wanted my son to be healthy and happy. Holding this image, it became clear what could help us achieve it. We needed to change his diet to help his digestion; we needed to increase his movement to improve his breathing; and we needed to develop and nourish his hobbies to elevate his happiness. When this became clear, with some thinking, research, advice, and experiments, I was able to pinpoint the specific methods that suited our needs and integrate them into our daily routine, our *Dinacharya*. With time, the more I practiced each method, the more I could go deeper and truly understand its benefits on the mental, emotional, and physical levels.

So now it's your turn. Hold your wishful image in your mind's eye. Recall all of its aspects, and try to answer the following questions with the intention of finding the method that can help you manifest your image:

- **Body** – What kind of body does the man/woman I wish to become have, and what can help me achieve this healthy body I envision?

- **Mind** – What kind of thoughts does the man/woman I wish to become have, and what can help me achieve the kind of thoughts I wish to have?

- **Emotions** – What kind of emotions does the man/woman I wish to become have, and what can help me feel the emotions I wish to have?

- **Giving (Out)** – What would the man/woman I wish to become be giving, and what can help me create and produce what I wish to offer to the world?

- **Behavior** – What kind of behavior does the man/woman I wish to become have, and what can help me improve my behavior in different situations to match that which I am contemplating upon?

- **Receiving (In)** – What does the man/woman I wish to become receive from life as direct feedback to who she/he is, and what can help me be more open to receiving and being deserving of these gifts?

Really stop for a few minutes and think about this. This process may take time, and repetition is an important step for this to really work.

This process of charting your method or action list to follow is the vehicle that will bring you to your destination. If you receive an answer, great! Write it down. If nothing comes up yet, simply mark this question and return to it after doing a bit of research on the topic.

You don't have to focus on all of these categories at the same time. Try to find one or two methods you believe are most important for you. The trick is to find the one method that you believe will help you achieve all of these aspects simultaneously.

Now, when you're ready, you can move on to the next step of charting your map.

Step 3: The Inspirational Story

The third step in creating your Storia Map is a short inspirational story. It is not enough to have an image and a list of methods; there should be a thread that ties it all together, a few sentences that touch your core value and integrate your methods into a coherent and meaningful story that describes the image of your new reality.

A story is like the *"Pran"*—the vital energy that flows in our body and connects us with something bigger than ourselves. The story connects us to our imagination, emotion, and our personal history. It connects us to other people and to our shared story in a beautiful dance of growth, evolution, and diversity.

Eventually, your Storia Map can resemble the imprint of your soul on this beautiful world we are a part of and on all the people you have touched and influenced in a positive and meaningful way.

When we construct our inspirational story, it is a gift for our soul, a boost to our strength and resilience. This creates a place of peace where our nervous system can go back to the "rest and digest" state in which the parasympathetic nervous system becomes more active, moving away from the fight-or-flight of the sympathetic nervous system. The inspirational story can do all that if you choose a story that:

1. Stimulates your hopes and imagination for a balanced, fulfilled life.

2. Gives you inner power to stand your ground and live out your truth.

3. Supports you and promotes confidence by giving you a reference that reminds you again and again that your goal is achievable because you or somebody else have already achieved something similar before.

Your story might be comprised of small and personal but significant events that had an impact on who you are, the deeper part of you, your soul, your Atman. You don't have to mention where you were born, where you lived and worked. It's not a résumé but a reminder of your core values and beliefs, a way to communicate (internally and externally) who you truly are and what you came to do on this earth.

Throughout the years, I collected many stories for my personal "inspirational story library." These stories are a reference to me on how I can be in various circumstances. My favorite inspirational stories are those that are based on true events, with people like you and me that have changed and transformed their lives and the lives of others for the better.

One such story is *Dolphin Tale*. This is a book that was also made into a film, inspired by the true story about a young dolphin that lost her tail after becoming entangled in a rope attached to a crab trap, followed by her rescue off the Florida coast. She was taken to the Clearwater Marine Aquarium, where she was named "Winter" and learned how to swim without a tail. The story develops more when Winter's life is threatened because of the pressure on her spine as a result of her altered swimming motion. To heal her, the first-ever prosthetic tail was designed. She was now challenged with learning how to swim with the prosthetic tail, which she did. Winter became a hero figure and a role model for hundreds of thousands around the world. Children and adults with prosthetics from all over the world came to see her.

Other inspirational stories I gathered are fictional stories, but they are also very motivational and powerful, like *The NeverEnding Story,* for example. I also drew some inspirational stories from the Bible and the New Testament, like the story of David and Goliath, where a young boy defeats the mighty giant, or the story of the brave and compassionate Mary, mother of Jesus, who, through her faith and devotion to God, helped to bring the child of God into the world, overcoming many threats and challenges.

Other inspirational stories that I use in Arieldavid's and my own Storia Maps come from Hinduism, Judaism, and Buddhism. I also take a lot of inspiration from novels such as *Siddhartha*, written in 1922 by German writer Hermann Hesse. This novel deals with the spiritual journey of self-discovery of a man named Siddhartha.

In Arieldavid's Storia Map, we have constructed short stories in the form of mantras, which we recite at the end of our daily practice and before going to bed. At the end of our daily practice, we look at the portrait of his future self, painted by Massimo, and I describe the story behind it, emphasizing how healthy and strong Arieldavid is, traveling the world with his family, sharing his story with others.

Before going to bed, we recite an additional aspect of his story: "Arieldavid is a chief, riding a horse. Arieldavid is strong, independent, and connected to himself and the environment." These short mantras incorporate the key elements of his inspirational story of independence, giving to the world, and his love for horses.

Take the time to think about your own inspirational stories, and you will see that you already have a vast collection of them; stories that guide your beliefs and decisions and act as role models to how you want to live your life. Use them as examples to build your own personal story. As I mentioned in the beginning of this section, your story should make you feel empowered, hopeful, and happy. You should keep it alive by reshaping it, developing it, and returning to it as frequently as possible, preferably once a day during your Storia Map meditation.

Step 4: The Sigil

Now we have our image, which, like a lighthouse, illuminates our destination. Now we have our method, which, like a ship, brings us closer to our destination day by day. Now we have our story, which guides our efforts and gives us reason and strength to move on, like the wind in our sails. We are finally ready to put it all together in a coherent visual representation of our journey—a map. But this is not an ordinary map; this is the Storia Map. It doesn't only show us the way to our destination; it magically pulls us toward it. And for it to have magical properties, it needs to be a sigil. To create a sigil, we first must choose a symbol. This symbol should hold special meaning for you.

For Arieldavid's Storia Map, as well as my own, I chose the hexagram symbol, also known as the Star of David—two triangles that overlap, one facing up and the other facing down. This is a very powerful ancient symbol with very deep meaning and is used in different traditions and cultures throughout the history of mankind. One of those uses is a representation of the heart chakra, which according to *Bhrigu* yoga, is the seat of strength for creation itself.

Now that you have chosen your special symbol comes the creative part. Take a pen and paper and draw the symbol. Try to make it precise and aesthetic but also playful and fun to look at. Feel free to add some colors and any other creative attributes that you might think of.

Now recall your image, method, and story. Choose key words, colors, and other symbols that might represent them, and incorporate them into the symbol. This is the most crucial part, so take your time and have fun with it. The result should be an artwork that makes you proud and excites you, not necessarily because it is objectively beautiful but because it holds your essence, your core values, your deepest aspirations. Because it reconnects you with your higher self and shows you the way to the world you wish to manifest. And because it reminds you that you are the narrator of your own life's story, a magician, a sorcerer of your reality.

Congratulations! If you have followed all the instructions, you should now have your first Storia Map, and you can begin your magical journey, knowing that you are on the right path.

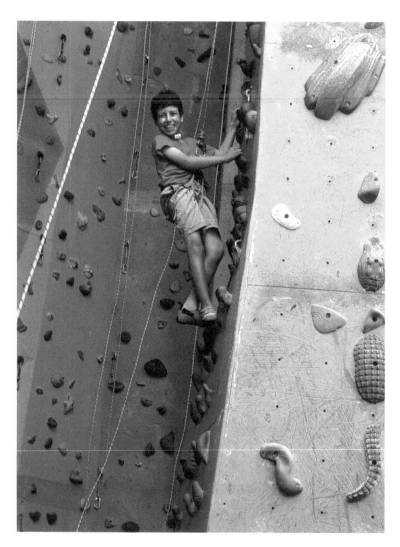

Arieldavid at Gecko Climbing Wall, 2018

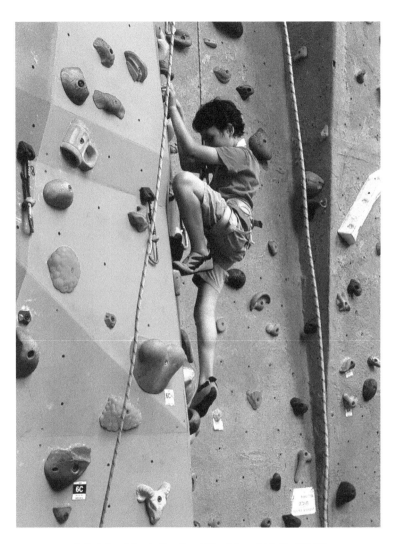

Arieldavid at Gecko Climbing Wall, 2018

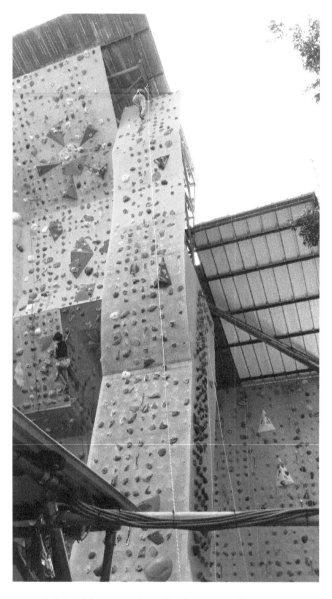

*Arieldavid at Gecko Climbing Wall, climbing
17-meter-high wall, 2018*

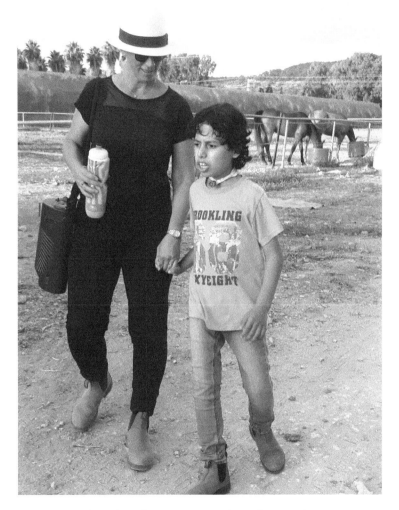

Arieldavid and Yamina at Gizmo's Ranch, 2019

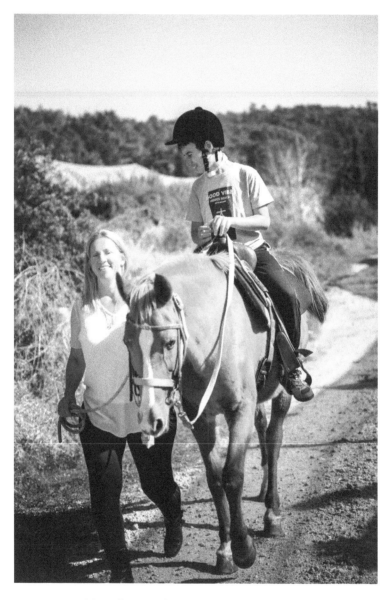

Arieldavid Horseback Riding with Yamina at
Gizmo's Ranch, 2020

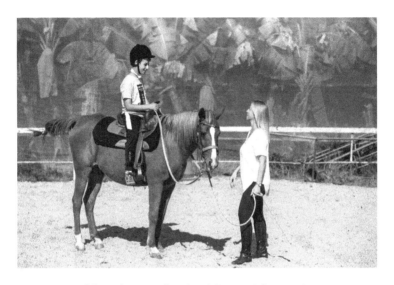

Arieldavid Horseback Riding with Yamina at Gizmo's Ranch, 2020

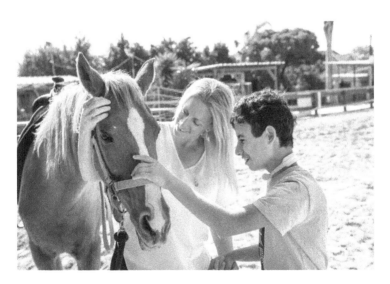

Arieldavid and Yamina at Gizmo's Ranch, 2020

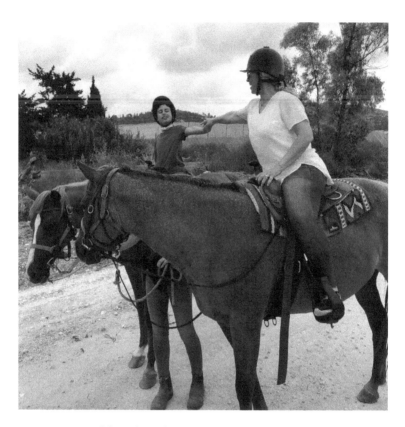

Arieldavid and Yamina at Gizmo's Ranch,
Horseback Riding together, side by side, 2020

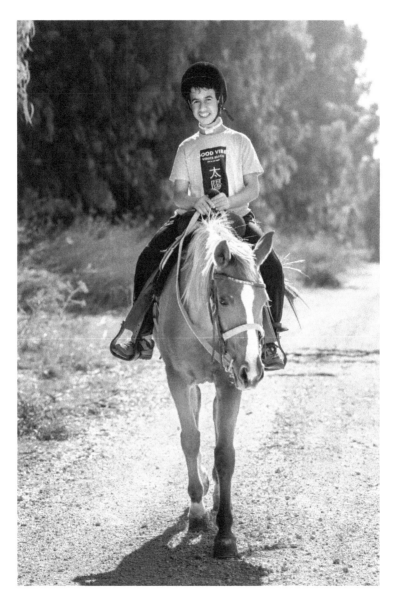

Arieldavid Horseback Riding at Gizmo's Ranch, 2020

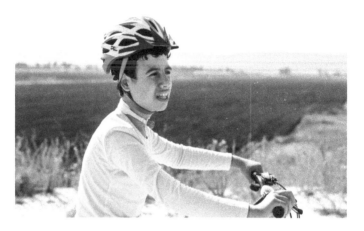

Arieldavid and Yamina bicycling together, 2020

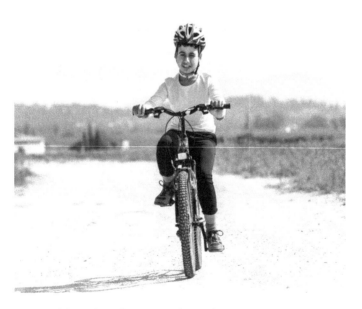

Arieldavid and Yamina bicycling together, 2020

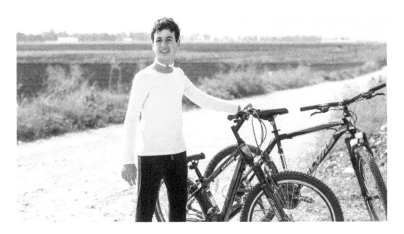

Arieldavid and Yamina bicycling together, 2020

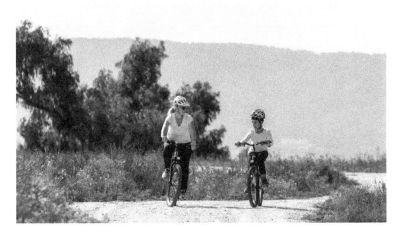

Arieldavid and Yamina bicycling together
side by side, 2020

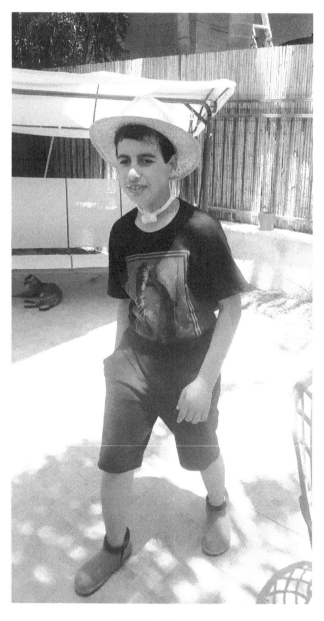

Arieldavid, 2021

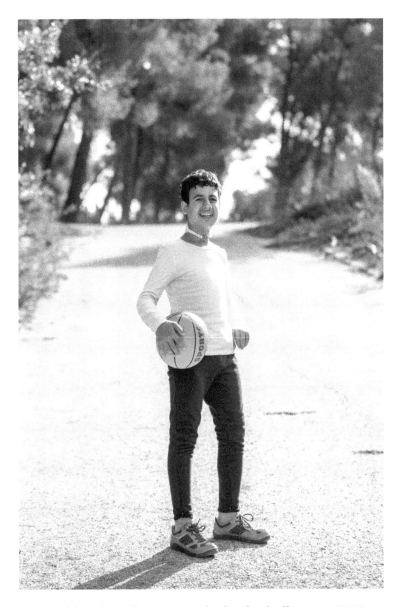

Arieldavid on the way to the basketball court, 2020

The Storia Map

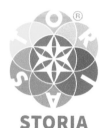

STORIA

Overview: Like in the tale of Fatima, we embarked on a long journey together and hopefully learned a few things and gained a few tools. Now that our journey is ending and you are beginning your own Storia Map journey, it's time to put all of our new knowledge to use and "build a tent for the emperor." Or in other words, to chart your own map to reach your higher self. Return to the Tree Meditation to reconnect with your core value. Return to the My Life's Exhibition exercise to recall the meaningful events that shaped your life's story. Return to the Farmer's Meditation and recall the Good Seeds you wish to plant in the fields of your subconscious mind. Holding all of this in your mind, you are now looking at the better version of yourself—at your higher self. Let's paint the portrait of this amazing person that you're looking at, so you can always be in touch with him or her:

Steps

1. The Wishful Image

    Using your imagination, good intentions, and all of the other tools at your disposal, construct an image of your Higher Self, of the reality you wish for yourself and others. Make this image as vivid and detailed as possible as you describe its different aspects to yourself:

- **Body** – What does your body look like? How does it feel?

- **Mind** – What are your thoughts like? Their quality? Their direction? Their subject?

- **Emotions** – What emotions visit you most frequently?

- **Behavior** – How does the person you wish to become behave in different situations?

- **Giving (Out)** – What are you able to create and give to the world?

- **Receiving (In)** – What gifts do you receive from the world?

2. The Practical Method

Now that you have a clear picture of where you're going, ask yourself how you want to get there:

- **Body** – What can help you achieve this healthy body you envision?

- **Mind** – What can help you achieve the kinds of thoughts you wish to have?

- **Emotions** – What can help you feel the emotions you wish to host?

- **Behavior** – What can help you improve your behavior in different situations?

- **Giving (Out)** – What can help you create and produce what you wish to offer to the world?

- **Receiving (In)** – What can help you be more open to receiving gifts from the world?

3. The Inspirational Story

A good story gives us structure and guides our beliefs and decisions. It inspires and motivates us. Recall the meaningful events from your past and the meaningful experiences you wish to have in the future. Now, recall the stories that had a strong, positive impact throughout your life, and use their essence to write your own epic story where you are the hero and life is your tale.

- **Body** – Which story inspires your body to be healthy?

- **Mind** – Which story inspires your mind to learn and develop?

- **Emotions** – Which story inspires you to balance and strengthen your emotions?

- **Behavior** – Which story inspires you to behave like the hero you wish to become?

- **Giving (Out)** – Which story inspires you to create and give to the world?

- **Receiving (In)** – Which story inspires you to be open to receiving life's presents?

4. The Sigil

    Now let's put it all together:

    a. Choose a sigil, a special symbol that you relate to, and draw it on a big piece of paper. Try to make it aesthetic but also fun and colorful.

    b. Review your answers from the previous sections and try to convert them into small visual representations that capture the essence of these answers. For example, a key word, a short sentence, a symbol, a color, a small drawing, and so on.

    c. Now take these key words and symbols that represent the different aspects of your higher self and arrange them inside the sigil. Take your time and have fun with it. The more time and creativity you put in, the more powerful your sigil will become.

    d. When you're satisfied with the result, you can stop for a moment and marvel at your new creation. Congratulations! You now have your own personal Storia Map, which means that you are all set to begin your journey toward your higher self. You can frame your Storia Map and put it in an accessible place that holds meaning for you. Once a day, look at your map to draw power from it and remind yourself where you are headed. Good luck!

If you're not sure where to begin, you can always use the original template of the Storia Map:

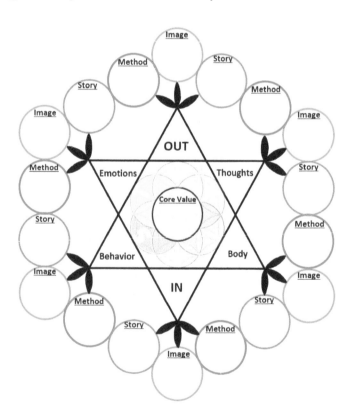

EPILOGUE
Bringing a Hug to the World

*UNLESS someone like you cares a whole awful lot,
nothing is going to get better, it's not.*

–Dr. Seuss

At the beginning of this book, I shared with you one of my favorite stories—the tale of Fatima, who lost everything and ultimately gained happiness and fulfillment by piecing everything she learned together in order to help others fulfill their dreams. During my quest to heal my son, I, too, have lost many things, and like Fatima, I have also gained a lot through my journey. Throughout this book, I shared with you the things I have gained, the tools that worked for me along the way in hopes that they will serve you and help you create the life you wish to manifest.

I would like to complete this book by sharing with you another story, a profound experience I had in 2008, when Arieldavid was three years old, while I was studying *guarire* (healing energy) in a little chapel in Le Case, near the Middle Ages city of Assisi. This experience forever changed my life and the way I look at my own destiny.

The *guarire* teaching took place in a small chapel in the mountains of Umbria. For three days we chanted, sang, meditated, and prayed. The teaching was done by Mr. F, a master of *guarire* who was guided directly by Mr. Paoletti.

On my second day in the morning, I was very emotional and was praying intensely for my son's health. After I prayed, I opened my eyes and quietly gazed upon a simple and elegant small statue of Mary, mother of Jesus, that was standing in the front of the chapel not far from where I sat.

It was a statue that was somewhat typical to the area of Assisi. Mary was dressed in a simple garment in the color of royal blue; her palms were facing out by her thighs. When I closed my eyes to meditate, I felt a warmth in my heart that began to spread all over my body. Suddenly, in my mind's eye, I saw the statue of Mary come to life. I saw Mary standing right next to me. She bent toward me and gave me a big hug. Her whole body wrapped mine, and I felt safe, calm, and empowered by her pure energy of love. It felt so good. There were no thoughts of how this was even possible. Only happiness and gratitude filled my mind.

When I finally got up from my meditation, I headed out of the chapel for lunch. While exiting the chapel, Mr. F turned to me. "What did you just see?" he asked me.

I was not keen to share this story. I was afraid he would think I had gone mad. And so I just said, "I would rather not talk about it."

But Mr. F was persistent. "You saw Mary just now, didn't you? She came to you and hugged you. Is that right?"

I was stunned. How could he possibly know that? Bewildered and amazed, I nodded my head and softly said, "Yes, that is exactly what happened." Still mesmerized by this magical moment, I felt gratitude and relief, as it assured me that what I had experienced was not imaginary.

"Bring this hug to the world," he said and smiled.

With this book I attempt to do just that, with hopes that it will help you see that no matter who you are, what you have been through, or what you are still going through, we are all always capable of love. We can always do something with it. We can always improve our lives and the lives of the people around us.

May it be the smallest gesture, a smile, a hug, an optimistic thought, a good word . . . . They all add up! Just keep at it, never giving up on what's important. Every day, plant your seeds and water them, nourishing the story you want to tell the world, determined, but with no expectations. And before you know it, with God's grace, you'll find yourself standing in a marvelous garden enjoying the sweet fruits of your labor and hopefully sharing them with the world. I wish you all the best on your journey to becoming your best self. And always remember—no matter what your history is, the future is yet to be told.

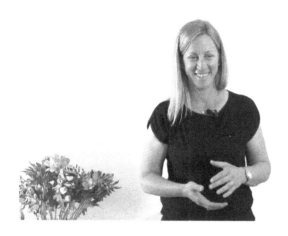

Yamina coaching at a Storia workshop, 2018

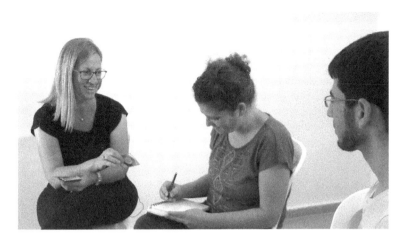

*Yamina coaching Naama and Liran with Storia cards
at a Storia workshop, 2018*

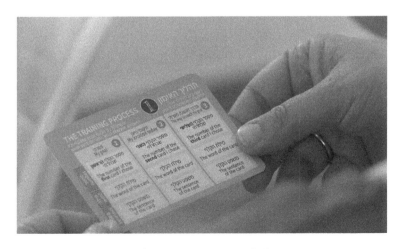

Storia cards at a Storia workshop, 2018

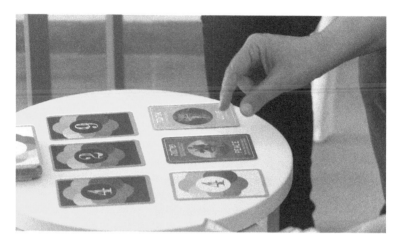

Storia cards at a Storia workshop, 2018

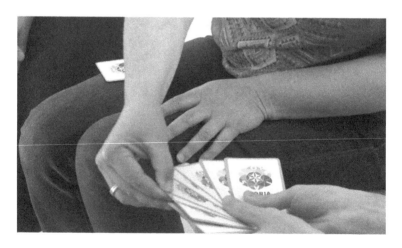

Storia cards at a Storia workshop, 2018

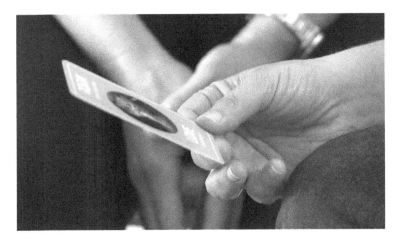

Storia cards at a Storia workshop, 2018

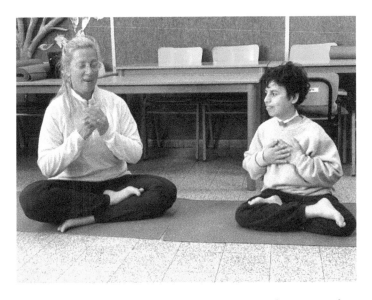

Arieldavid and Yamina teaching a yoga class together
to AD's classmates, Genigar School, 2019

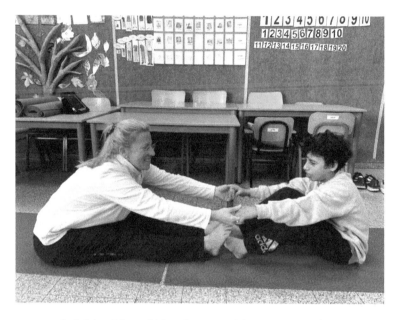

*Arieldavid and Yamina teaching a yoga class
together to AD's classmates, Genigar School, 2019*

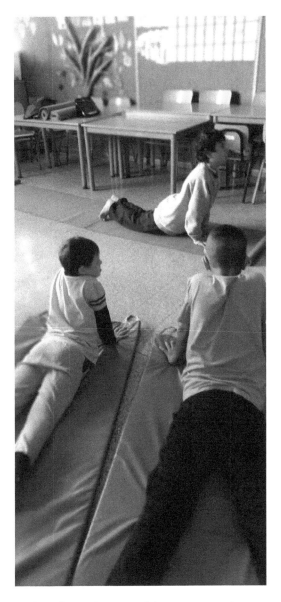

Arieldavid and Yamina teaching a yoga class together
to AD's classmates, Genigar School, 2019

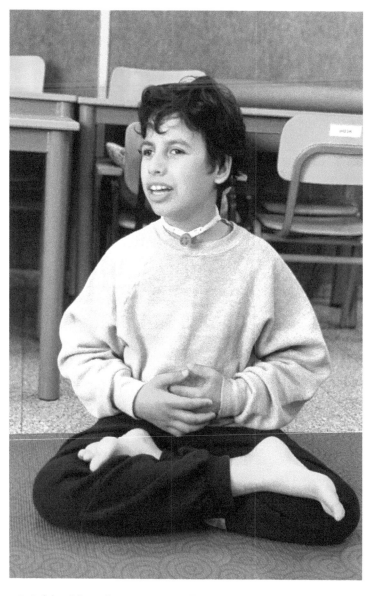

Arieldavid and Yamina teaching a yoga class together
to AD's classmates, Genigar School, 2019

Prayer Of St. Francis

Lord, make me an instrument of your peace;
where there is hatred, let me sow love;
where there is injury, pardon;
where there is doubt, faith;
where there is despair, hope;
where there is darkness, light;
and where there is sadness, joy.

O Divine Master,
grant that I may not so much seek to be consoled
as to console;
to be understood, as to understand;
to be loved, as to love;
for it is in giving that we receive,
it is in pardoning that we are pardoned,
and it is in dying that we are born to Eternal Life.

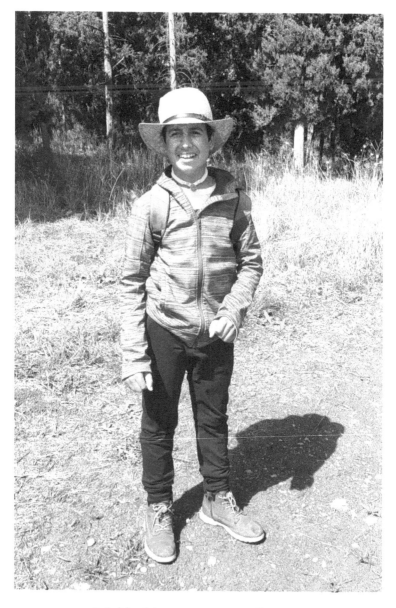

Arieldavid on a nature walk, 2021

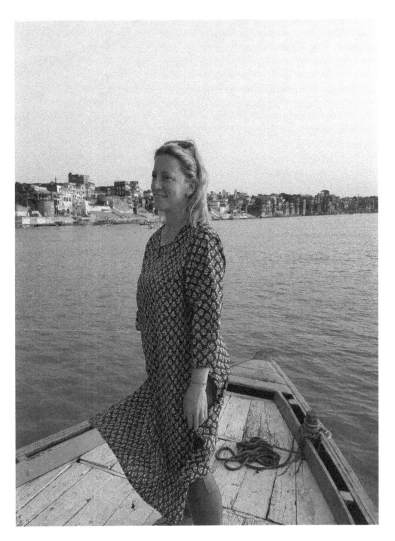

Yamina visiting the River Ganges/Maa Ganga
during a Bhrigu yoga workshop, Varanasi, 2019

References

- Bhadury, Dr. J.K. (2001). *Sermon About Yoga*. Bhrigu Publications, Ramapura, Varanasi, India.

- Brunton, P. (2003). *A Search in Secret India: The Classic Work on Seeking a Guru*. Ebury Press.

- D. Dyer, W.W. (2004). *The Power of Intention: Learning to Co-Create Your World Your Way*. Hay House.

- Frankl, E.V. *Man's Search for Meaning*. (1959). Beacon Press.

- Iyengar, B.K.S. *Light on Life*. (2020). HarperCollins Publishers/Yellow Kite.

- Lad, Dr. V. (1984). *Ayurveda, The Science of Self-Healing*. Lotus press.

- Lad, Dr. V. (2012). *Textbook of Ayurveda, General Principles of Management and Treatment, Volume 3*. Albuquerque, New Mexico: The Ayurvedic Press.

- Lipton, H.B. (2016). *The Biology of Belief 10th Anniversary Edition: Unleashing the Power of Consciousness, Matter and Miracles*. Hay House.

- Neville, (1952) (2012), *The Power of Awareness*, Jeremy P. Tarcher/Penguin.

- Ouspensky, P.D. (1949). *In Search of the Miraculous: Fragments of an Unknown Teaching.* The Library of Alexandria.

- Rollins, J.A., Bolig R., and Mahan, C.C. (2005). *Meeting Children's Psychological Needs, Across the Health Care Continuum.* Austin: PRO-ED.

- Shah, I. (1967). *Tales of the Dervishes.* Dutton and Co.

- Stewart, A. (2019). *Yoga as Self-Care for Health-Care Practitioners, Cultivating Resilience, Compassion and Empathy.* Singing Dragon.

- Stiles, M. (2002) (interpreted). *Yoga Sutras of Patanjali.* Weiser Books.

- Sri Swami Satchidananda. (1978). *The Yoga Sutras of Patanjali – Translation and Commentary.* International Yoga Publications. Buckingham, Virginia.

- Sullivan, M., and Hyland Robertson. C. (2020). *Understanding Yoga Therapy, Applied Philosophy and Science for Health and Well-Being.* New York: Routledge.

- Thoreau, H.D. (1854) (2012). *Walden.* Empire Books.

- Tiwari, M. (1995). *A Life of Balance: The Complete Guide to Ayurvedic Nutrition and Body Types with Recipes.* Healing Arts Press.

- Wattles, D.W. (2007). *The Science of Getting Rich, The Proven Mental Program to a Life of Wealth.* Tarcher Perigee.

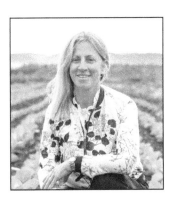

This is Yamina Salomon's debut. Yamina is a mother, wife, and creator of the "Storia Map" method developed for her son, Arieldavid, to create the life she envisioned for him against all odds. She is a Storia meditation teacher, certified yoga teacher, Bhrigu yoga practitioner, holds a BFA from Parsons School of Design (New York), and an MFA from Domus Academy (Milan, Italy). After her son was born, Yamina devoted herself to his healing and development. Today, Yamina offers her knowledge to others for spiritual growth and to facilitate their healing path.

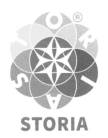

STORIA

To get in touch with Yamina and learn about her lectures, Storia Map workshops, and individual sessions, please visit Yamina's website, WWW.STORIAMAP.COM, or email her at yamina@storiamap.com.